7/2015

Bridging the Gap

How Community Health Workers Promote the Health of Immigrants

SALLY E. FINDLEY

SERGIO E. MATOS

OXFORD
UNIVERSITY PRESS

Oxford University Press is a department of the University of
Oxford. It furthers the University's objective of excellence in research,
scholarship, and education by publishing worldwide.

Oxford   New York
Auckland   Cape Town   Dar es Salaam   Hong Kong   Karachi
Kuala Lumpur   Madrid   Melbourne   Mexico City   Nairobi
New Delhi   Shanghai   Taipei   Toronto

With offices in
Argentina   Austria   Brazil   Chile   Czech Republic   France   Greece
Guatemala   Hungary   Italy   Japan   Poland   Portugal   Singapore
South Korea   Switzerland   Thailand   Turkey   Ukraine   Vietnam

Oxford is a registered trademark of Oxford University Press
in the UK and certain other countries.

Published in the United States of America by
Oxford University Press
198 Madison Avenue, New York, NY 10016

Library of Congress Cataloging-in-Publication Data
Findley, Sally E., author
Bridging the gap : how community health workers promote the health of immigrants / Sally E. Findley
and Sergio E. Matos.
p. ; cm.
ISBN 978-0-19-936432-9
I. Matos, Sergio E., author.   II. Title
[DNLM: 1. Emigrants and Immigrants—United States.   2. Community Health Workers—United
States.   3. Health Promotion—United States.   4. Health Status Disparities—United States.
WA 300 AA1]
RA448.5.I44
362.1086'912—dc23
2014046434

9 8 7 6 5 4 3 2 1
Printed in the United States of America
on acid-free paper

Contents

Foreword

TO EXPAND IMMIGRANT ACCESS TO HEALTH CARE, COMMUNITY IS KEY

Nisha Agarwal and Sam Solomon

WE LIVE IN an era of remarkable nationwide expansion of access to health insurance—likely the greatest such expansion since the implementation of Medicaid, and rivaling or even surpassing the effect of the Children's Health Insurance Program. The Patient Protection and Affordable Care Act of 2010 (ACA), according to the latest estimates, will expand health insurance coverage to 26 million uninsured individuals over the next decade. In New York City, after just the first year of open enrollment by the state's health insurance exchange, experts have estimated that the number of 1.1 million or so uninsured New York City residents declined by as much as 45%.

Without diminishing the accomplishments of the ACA—the exchanges, subsidies, Medicaid expansion, insurance regulations, and more—it is also important to recognize what the ACA does *not* accomplish. This era of expansion has proceeded apace without a significant segment of our population: millions upon millions of immigrants, both undocumented and many of those with status. Undocumented immigrants are specifically excluded from purchasing health insurance plans and receiving federal subsidies through the ACA's insurance exchanges, as are recipients of deferred action, including the 700,000-plus recipients of the Deferred Action for Childhood Arrivals (DACA) program and the millions more deferred action recipients to come in the wake of the 2014 administrative reforms. These exclusions are rooted in precedent. Federal and state exclusions render deferred-action recipients in most states ineligible for Medicaid and CHIP, other than for treatment of emergency conditions. (New York, thanks to the Child Health Plus program enacted in 1990, provides government-subsidized health insurance to undocumented children, as do several other states.) The 1996 welfare reform law authorizes states to exclude lawful immigrants from their Medicaid programs for a period of 5 years after their arrival. Many employers, especially of low-wage immigrant workers, do not offer affordable employer-sponsored insurance plans. As a result of all these factors and more, many undocumented and lawfully present immigrants remain without access to health insurance, with uninsurance rates among noncitizen immigrants at nearly 50%. Despite the health-policy truism that insurance is no guarantee of access, uninsurance and unaffordability are clearly among the largest contributors to the problems faced by immigrants seeking access to basic health care.

Immigrant access to care also faces other barriers: insufficient language access, cultural norms, geographic inaccessibility, fear of interaction with government institutions, fear of discrimination, misconceptions about "public charge" grounds for inadmissibility, and limited health literacy and health insurance literacy, among others. Alongside insurance eligibility exclusions, these barriers leave governments and community organizations with a range of continuing challenges to ensure immigrant access to care.

As Sally Findley and Sergio Matos make clear in *Bridging the Gap*, the key to addressing these challenges is community-level support. Community-based health care navigation, provided by community health workers (CHWs) and others, is of particularly vital importance to immigrant communities for a number of reasons—the trust that community members have for local providers, the ability to communicate in their native language, and the welcoming environment of the familiar. But perhaps the most important of those reasons is that community-based support communicates an invaluable message: "You are not alone." This is the message of one of the many CHWs and community members whose voices are included in *Bridging the Gap*, and it is a powerful message. Among immigrant populations who are marginalized and excluded from many parts of the mainstream economy, that message—"You are not alone"—can make all the difference in seeking care for their chronic condition or gaining access to immunizations for their child. That difference is real and quantifiable; community integration and social connectedness are strong determinants of health, as has been repeatedly demonstrated in research on overall mortality rates, heart disease, depression, and other conditions. Community-based support for health care access—the work done by CHWs and others—saves lives.

The need for community-based support is most acute in the area of access to primary and preventive care. It is in these areas that immigrants' high rate of uninsurance and lack of access to ongoing medical care are most harmful, resulting in a long-term public health crisis—evidence of which is apparent from the well-documented erosion of the "healthy migrant" effect over immigrants' life spans. Findley and Matos do not mince words: "The lack of preventive or routine care increases the chance that the early signs of illness will be missed, and treatment may only be sought when the condition reaches an advanced stage requiring intensive and often costly intervention." The implications for public health, health insurance, immigration law, and economics are profound. With broad-based policy solutions having proven politically elusive in many places across the United States, community-based supports like CHWs are an absolute necessity.

Bridging the Gap points a way forward to support immigrant health access at the height of a period of rancorous debates in both health care and immigration. Findley and Matos provide the knowledge, the analysis, and the practical tools to improve immigrant health access, despite the challenges posed by exclusions and acrimony. Drawing focus to the old-fashioned but undeniably effective modalities of shoe leather and community engagement, Findley and Matos have produced a guide to CHW implementation that will be of enormous importance to community-based organizations, health care providers, public health officials, and the governmental and academic health policy communities.

Nisha Agarwal (J.D., Harvard Law School) is the Commissioner of New York City Mayor's Office of Immigrant Affairs.

Sam Solomon (J.D., Benjamin N. Cardozo School of Law) is a Policy Analyst for New York City Mayor's Office of Immigrant Affairs.

Acknowledgments

MANY PEOPLE HAVE helped to shape our thinking and our commitment to *Bridging the Gap*. This book contains both shared and individual experiences of the coauthors, who have been colleagues for over 20 years. In a sense, the seeds for the book were planted when Sally was mentored by Sidney Goldstein in the 1980s at Brown University, where he encouraged her to probe deeply beneath the surface to hear migrants' stories, to understand the inequities driving migrant choices and in turn how migration brought fundamental changes to their own lives and those of their families and communities. At the end of 1990s we met and began working together to strengthen community health worker programs in Northern Manhattan and elsewhere in New York. The book began in early 2000s when we both realized that the community health worker (CHW) story we had to tell was much bigger than the individual articles we might write when reporting on a project. We recognized that the stories of caring, love, courage, and heroism we were experiencing in our work with CHWs had to be told. Our dream to think on a larger scale was encouraged by Jacqueline Martinez Garcel, first while she was the director of the Northern Manhattan Community Voices Collaborative and then when she joined the New York State Health Foundation and supported our work to advance CHWs in New York State. We also thank other partners in the Northern Manhattan Community Voices Collaborative, Thelma Adair, Mario Drummonds, Walid Michelen, and Moises Perez, who challenged us to consider different ways that CHWs could be integrated into community health programs. Members of the CHW Network of NYC board of directors, particularly Bakary Tandia at African Services Committee, were very supportive to us as we developed our ideas. Within the American Public Health Association CHW Section membership, we are much indebted to Hector Balcazar, Noelle Wiggins, Susan Mayfield-Johnson,

Lee Rosenthal, and Lisa Renee Holderby Fox. Several partners in the Start Right and Asthma Basics for Children coalitions in New York City contributed immeasurably to the success of our strategies and to our understanding of what things could work well for immigrants, notably Maria Lizardo, Kelly Lubeck, Miriam Mejia, Patricia Peretz, Martha Sanchez, and Gloria Thomas. Our friends and colleagues at the New York University Langone Medical School Prevention Research Center, Chau Trinh-Shevrin, Nadia Islam, Mariano Rey, and Smiti Kapadia-Nadkarni, contributed their extensive experiences working with CHWs in immigrant communities to this work. We both learned a great deal from April Hicks, whose sharp questions helped us stay focused on CHW workforce development strategies that truly engage and empower CHWs. We are indebted to several graduate students and research assistants who helped with the many interviews that went into the *Bridging the Gap* story: Flor Camerena, Nirshila Chand, Tener Huang, Brian Johnson, Megan Larkin, Rosa Madera-Reese, and Constanza Tobasio. In the international arena, conversations with colleagues Fatima Adamu, Godwin Afenyadu, Seydou Doumbia, and Eric Swedberg helped us make the connections between CHW work in New York and West Africa. We are also deeply grateful to the many CHWs from the independent nations of the Organization of Eastern Caribbean States who contributed their passion as CHWs to the realization of this book, particularly Dennis James and Deborah Williams from the Republic of Trinidad and Tobago.

We have worked with hundreds of CHWs over the years, and all the stories shared here have impacted our lives and pushed us to publish this work. We thank them all. But among the many stories of CHW bravery and fortitude in the face of unimaginable challenges, Romelia Corvacho's story stands out as what drove us to begin and continue this work. We thank her for inspiring us to undertake this adventure.

As important as all these people have been to shaping our thinking, this book would never have happened had it not been for the respite and inspiration afforded by a month-long residency awarded to Sally by the Rockefeller Foundation Bellagio Center. After years of work on multiple projects, all competing simultaneously for attention, to have one month dedicated solely to this book made all the difference in the world. We are particularly grateful to Rob Garris, director of the Bellagio Center Programs, who supported this work before, during, and after her Bellagio residency.

The guiding star to whom we owe the biggest thanks is Sally's late husband, Richard Glass, who encouraged her to weave this story together into the book that it has become. It is in his memory that we dedicate this book.

December 2014
Sally Findley and Sergio E. Matos

Introduction

IN THE WINTER of 2006 at a small child care program in Washington Heights, New York City a timid young Mexican immigrant sat down at a special parents' workshop we were hosting on asthma, which was led in Spanish by a young Dominican immigrant. As the mother listened, it dawned on her that her young child's repeated colds and flus might be asthma, not colds, as the doctor in Mexico had told her before she came north. After the program was over, she came up to speak with the workshop leader about her child's repeated illnesses. The workshop leader discovered that the child had already been to the emergency department twice because of these breathing problems, which means that the child's illness—if it was asthma—was fairly serious. She invited the mother to participate in a program we offered to help parents learn how to manage their child's asthma, and the mother promptly enrolled. Through this program she started on the path to helping her child become well: signing the child up for health insurance, going to the doctor and learning that the child indeed had asthma, and then learning how to take care of her child and her home so that the child did not suffer from repeated asthma attacks. As she said later,

> When we lived in Mexico, my child was always sick and I kept going to the doctor to get medicine. Our lives were changed by this program. With the help of the promotora, I was able to take my child to the doctor here and found out he had asthma. She [the promotora] helped me learn how to give my son the asthma medicine, and also how to keep him away from the dust that makes his asthma worse. I can't thank you enough.

This incident portrays the theme for this book, namely how community health workers (CHWs) help immigrants. The workshop leader was in fact a trained CHW, who worked with two dozen major day care or Head Start programs to help the children and parents at their centers gain control of asthma, which affected one in four of the children at these centers. The young mother was typical of many in this largely immigrant community, which included recent immigrants from Mexico, Ecuador, El Salvador, and the Dominican Republic. Like many immigrants, she did not have health insurance for herself, and she had been unaware that the New York child health insurance program is available for all children, regardless of their place of birth. Without the CHW, she and her child would have continued to suffer through multiple asthma attacks, nights in the emergency room, and missed days of child care.

Like immigrants in many cities in the United States and elsewhere, recent immigrants confront many challenges in coping with health issues. They may not speak the same language as the health care workers, making communication about the problem or its care very difficult. Even when they speak the same language, there may be cultural differences that make it hard for the immigrant to convey the problem or understand what is supposed to be done to prevent or cure it. In addition, the immigrant may not have a network of friends or family who can help him or her navigate the system. Added to all these social and cultural barriers is the financial barrier of health care. Recent immigrants are focused on getting jobs and saving to support their families. Health care comes as a luxury item, to be deferred unless absolutely necessary. Depending on how and where the immigrant does seek care, this can be extremely costly, as when the immigrant lacks insurance. Even when the immigrant might qualify for emergency health insurance subsidies, he or she may not know about or be willing to take advantage of these supports.

CHWs are uniquely positioned to help immigrant families with health issues. Typically, CHWs are from the community in which they work, and they may be immigrants themselves. They know the community, so they know where to find families in need of help with health problems, and because they are also members of that community, speaking the same language and sharing the same cultural traditions, they are welcome in immigrant homes. Many CHWs have themselves lived through similar difficulties, and they are able to help their fellow immigrants by sharing their experiences so that the instructions from the doctor are translated into practical, realistic steps that they can do. The CHW can help immigrants in obtaining health insurance or finding low-cost health care. Thus, in many ways, the CHW is critical in "bridging the gap" in both directions, helping bring immigrants to the health care system and then in translating the health care system recommendations back into the realities of the immigrants' world.

While much has been written about immigrant health, there has been relatively little that focuses on the processes by which immigrant families regain their health when it is challenged. In our two decades of work with immigrant families in New York City and across the United States, Africa and the Caribbean, we have observed the critical role CHWs play in this process. It has become apparent to us that CHWs are uniquely positioned to support the health needs and aspirations of immigrants. But, if you wanted to design a program for immigrants with CHWs, there is no book or guide to support you in developing such a program.

Hence, this book was conceived to fill that gap, to explain how CHWs have supported immigrants. It is informed by the work that we have been privileged to lead with almost 45,000 families and over 4,500 CHWs in Northern Manhattan, New York City, as well as with immigrants and CHWs in the Caribbean and West Africa, where both of us have worked. The outcomes of these activities have been reported previously in peer-reviewed manuscripts. (See several authored by Findley and/or Matos in the list of references at the end of the book.) Our purpose here is not to repeat those overall study findings but to focus on how the CHWs in these programs supported immigrant families, detailing how they were prepared as CHWs and what they did to help bridge the gap between the health system and immigrants. We tell the story of the coalitions using a combination of the outcome data and material collected as part of annual program feedback surveys, from 636 program participants and 102 CHWs in these programs. While the Northern Manhattan programs are central to this book's narrative, we have included material from the city, state, nation, and global situation in order to highlight the critical role played by CHWs in promoting the health of immigrant worldwide. This broader perspective is supported by material we collected with surveys conducted throughout New York State with 223 CHWs and 40 employers and nationally with in-depth telephone interviews with 53 immigrants and/ or CHWs and 8 CHW program managers, conducted as part of our long-term research into the development of training programs to advance CHWs in New York (CUMC IRB # AAAD0506). Our understanding of CHWs is further enhanced by our experience in building CHW programming in Africa and the Caribbean.

We begin our journey into the intersecting worlds of immigrants and CHWs by setting the global context, describing global immigration trends and then zooming in for a closer look at immigration patterns in the United

States. The immigration experience is widely varied, and part of the work of CHWs is to focus on the immigrants who are likely to have had the most turbulent and difficult migration experiences. While all foreign-born persons are technically immigrants, the greatest health differentials and therefore the greatest need for CHW support generally is among the most disadvantaged immigrant groups, those who do not speak English, have little or no formal education, and struggle, at least at first, to establish themselves in their new home and build a life for themselves and their family. Therefore, to set the stage, the first chapter introduces readers to global migration trends and immigrant health issues, illustrating these facts with the accounts of immigrants we have interviewed for this book.

Next, we introduce CHWs, outlining who they are and what they do. We present global and national statistics on CHWs, outlining the similarities in how CHWs work globally. This second chapter blends our in-depth knowledge of CHWs and their scope of practice in New York with evidence for their effectiveness in improving immigrant health from studies conducted throughout the United States and globally. It also includes a detailed review of the literature documenting how CHWs have supported improved health status for immigrants across diverse health problem areas.

The third chapter delves more deeply into how CHWs view their work with immigrants, using the findings from our surveys and in-depth interviews with New York State CHWs to tease out the attributes and activities that most contribute to CHWs' success with immigrants. Immigrants who choose to become CHWs are not like other immigrants. They have been tested by their immigration experience and have drawn on enormous well-springs of courage, perseverance, and energy to overcome threats and danger. Central to this chapter is to show how these immigrant experiences shape the desire, courage, and strengths of immigrant CHWs for work with and advocacy for other immigrants.

In the fourth chapter we explore more deeply into how CHWs have been incorporated into several programs in Northern Manhattan, New York City, where we have worked for the past two decades. It places this work in the context of the vibrant immigrant community of Washington Heights/Inwood, one of the city's leading immigrant destinations, and shows how community leaders advocated for CHWs as the central strategy for addressing the health needs of this immigrant community. The chapter integrates qualitative interviews and quantitative feedback surveys and programmatic evidence from three different coalitions to highlight how the programs' CHWs worked to support immigrant families in solving their health issues.

In the fifth chapter, we articulate three basic organizational structures for supporting CHWs in promoting immigrant health, incorporating discussions about programs in New York City and beyond to show how organizational structure may—underpin successful CHW programs for immigrants. The chapter gives examples of each type of program and uses published studies and additional in-depth interviews to illustrate the advantages and disadvantages of each organizational model for CHW programs focusing on immigrant health. The chapter also considers some hybrid models for CHW programming that blend elements of the three basic structures.

The book then closes with a return to the global perspective, drawing together the various lessons learned from the preceding chapters with a set of best-practice recommendations for strengthening CHW support for immigrant health, not just in New York but also in other large metropolitan areas where they concentrate. This perspective aims to fill a gap in our thinking about CHWs globally, which has tended to be informed by a view of CHWs as the barefoot doctors for underserved rural populations. Today and in the future, we will need CHWs who are adept at working in metropolitan settings and able to work across native and foreign-born populations.

1

Immigrant Health

IMMIGRATION TRENDS AND IMPACT ON HEALTH

Introduction

Throughout history, people have been on the move, both short and long distances. When asked about how long they have lived somewhere, one in five will have lived there only 5 years or less. While the majority of people who move do not go beyond the boundaries of their home country, a significant number do move to another country, whether forced by war or other circumstances as a refugee or voluntarily in pursuit of a better life. Unlike internal moves, these international moves are generally subject to visa or other entry requirements aimed at monitoring and/or regulating the flow of people into the host country. Like internal migrants, international migrants move in response to social, educational, and economic disparities and employment demand, as well as in response to political, economic, and climate-related crises. Thus, the past decades of political and economic change throughout the world have been accompanied by a rise in international migrants, referred to as immigrants, more than doubling in numbers between 1980 and 2010, from 100 to 214 million (United Nations Department of Economic and Social Affairs, 2011).

The enormity of the numbers of men, women, and children who are migrants today should not be taken as an indication that migration is an easy thing to do. Indeed, for most immigrants, it is often an arduous and risky process that can take years from the initial move to the final arrival at the planned destination, whether the move is from Africa to Sweden or from Central America to Oregon. For some, often young men and women who by choice, or, conversely, lack of any other choice, want to make it in the larger world, emigration may be staged, involving steps from village to nearby towns to the capital city, spending 1 or more years at each step earning enough money and building enough connections to make the next move. In some cases it takes several years before they are able to make the "big" move to their international destination (Massey, 1990). Others, perhaps more desperate to leave and start a new life in their chosen international destination, may expend their life savings or go heavily into debt simply to pay the passage for the one or two family members on whom they are willing to take a chance that they will indeed make it to the destination and manage to establish themselves there. Many are fleeing political persecution or violence (Findley, 2001). Thousands rely on traffickers or "coyotes," and there is no guarantee that they will make it, as evidenced by the many stories in the newspapers of waylaid boats, border walls unscaled, and detained or deported immigrants. In 2012 there were an estimated 20.9 million persons, mostly women and children, who were believed to be trafficked into forced labor (United Nations Department of Economic and Social Affairs, 2013). Yet, millions more become immigrants whose challenge begins after having arrived at their host countries as students, proceeding through a myriad of forms, applications, and barriers in pursuit of a work permit and eventual citizenship. Even those who are able legally to join other family members must wait a long time, with many hurdles to be cleared before the relatives are allowed to come (Castles, 2000, 2002; Massey, 2002, 2006). By whatever process, immigration in today's world is not for the meek. It takes courage, inner strength, perseverance, and single-minded focus on the goal of becoming an established and productive member of the host society.

The challenges, of course, are that by crossing into another country, the immigrant must pass through border controls, and these controls and their related enforcement agencies are designed to protect the nation's sovereign rights, not the human rights of the migrants themselves. Most evidence today suggests that immigrants contribute to the global economy and, in particular, to the US and European economies where millions head each yearly. (Hatton & Williamson, 2011). Almost all (91%) of the governments of more developed nations had policies promoting integration of nonnationals, and 39% had programs encouraging immigration of the highly skilled. Yet governments struggling to show that they are pro-jobs and doing everything they can to maintain full employment and keep taxes low typically opt for exclusionary policies that push back against irregular or undocumented immigrants. The majority of countries with the greatest number of irregular migrants (22 out of the 25) considered such migration a "major concern" (United Nations Department of Economic and Social Affairs, 2013).

In 2006, several initiatives were launched at the global level to enhance the benefits and address challenges associated with international migration, particularly irregular migration, beginning with a High-level Dialogue on International Migration and Development convened by the United Nations General Assembly. This dialogue recognized the inextricable linkages between migration, development, and human rights, and that an integrated approach is needed for both regular and irregular migration. The Global Migration Group established pursuant to this dialogue has now been meeting to develop and adopt coherent, comprehensive, and coordinated approaches to international migration. These efforts include conventions and protocols to prevent trafficking, especially of women and children, protection of refugees, and protection of the rights of all migrant workers and their families (United Nations Department of Economic and Social Affairs, 2011).

While there is now agreement that protecting the health of migrants is part of protecting their human right to health, the pathways to achieving that goal seem both long and fraught with difficulty. There is no Millennium Development Goal for immigrant health, and governments have by and large left immigrants to fend for themselves within the construct of national health policies and programs. The difficulty is that immigrants may not have equal access to this system, particularly if they are denied health insurance or benefits due to their immigration status. At the end of the day, immigrants know that they are responsible for their own health and that of their children, but if they do not have any health insurance coverage, are new to the community, or lack knowledge or resources to expend on medications or other prerequisites to a healthy life, they may not be able to sustain their health. Coming from settings with low chronic disease prevalence, they may be unfamiliar with asthma, diabetes, or hypertension, and therefore not likely to take steps to prevent these illnesses. Even if they have insurance, encounters with the health system may be disorienting and frustrating due to language or cultural barriers, entail additional costs beyond the limits of their income, and perhaps jeopardize their immigrant status, particularly if they fear deportation. Further, the very circumstances of their work, often in "3-D" jobs (dirty, difficult, dangerous), expose them to long hours, the chance of injury, and chronic health risks, such as cancer or other conditions related to toxic exposures (Lopez-Acuna, 2010). While global leaders may agree that health is a human right, we struggle to find approaches to promoting immigrant health that will work for the immigrants and for the host communities.

Part of addressing the problem is to be clear about the immigrants, their health issues, and which health concerns require a different approach, depending on how immigrants may or may not be lagging behind their compatriots, at home or in their new country. This chapter will provide an overview of global immigration trends and then zero in on immigration to the United States. We will then introduce several immigrants whom we have interviewed as part of the research for this book. We have selected these stories because they illustrate the different types of journeys, some more perilous than others, and the enormous resourcefulness needed to persist and succeed. Then, we will return to the issue of immigrant health, outlining the ways in which immigrants may face additional challenges to staying healthy. With our focus on community health workers, we will highlight the health problems that are susceptible to community health worker interventions. We will then return to the immigrant stories, to illustrate the challenges faced by the immigrants introduced at the beginning of the chapter. The chapter closes with a summary of the health issues faced by immigrants in the United States, particularly those who are undocumented and/or vulnerable, with low incomes and probably working in jobs without health insurance coverage, private or public.

Global Immigrant Trends

The pace of international migration quickened in the past decade, from 2000 to 2010, when their numbers increased from 179 to 214 million. Between 2005 and 2010 an average of 2.7 million persons per year immigrated to another country than their birth country. If all the immigrants were considered a country, it would be the fifth largest in the world. The more developed world hosted 60% of all the immigrants or foreign-born persons, with 10 countries accounting for 52% of all global immigrants: the United States with 20% of all immigrants, Russia with 6%, Germany with 5%, Saudi Arabia, Canada, France, United Kingdom, and Spain each with 3%, and India and Ukraine each with 2.5%. Between 2000 and 2010, 23% of the new global immigrants went to the United States, 13% to Spain, 7% to Italy, 6% to Saudi Arabia, and 5% each to the United Kingdom and Canada. Regardless of where the immigrants ended up, more had been born in the developing world than in the developed world. In 2010, 57% of the immigrants in the developed world were born in the developing world. If the same patterns continue, the total global population in 2050 is expected to be 404 million, with immigrants contributing 60 million to the total world population (United Nations Department of Economic and Social Affairs, 2011).

The rapid rise in immigrants reflects the essential role that immigrants play in the globalization of the economy, and immigration has moved to the top of national and international development agendas. We have now entered the migration decades, with labor migrations reinforcing the global economic ties between nations. Migration is essential for some societies to compensate for demographic trends and skill shortages, while for others the remittances are critical to national development.

The United States as a Major Destination for the World's Migrants

The United States leads all other countries in its number of immigrants, 42.8 million in 2010, accounting for 13.5% of the total US population. In 2009, just over half (51.8%) came from the following countries: Mexico (14.8%), China (5.7%), the Philippines (5.3%), India (5.1%), the Dominican Republic (4.4%), and the following with 3.5% or less: Cuba, Colombia, Haiti, South Korea, Jamaica, Pakistan, and Vietnam. The vast majority of foreign-born in the United States are from Mexico, which accounted for 11.5 million foreign-born, followed by 5.2 million from China, 4.5 million from the Philippines, 4.3 million from India, and 3 million or less from all other countries combined (Batalova & Lee, 2014).

In the United States, immigrants are concentrated along the coasts, border areas, and "ports of entry." (See Fig. 1.1.) These new immigrants went to the same group of states that already had large shares of immigrants: California (20.2%), New York (13.3%), Florida (11.2%), Texas (8.4%), New Jersey (5.2%), Illinois (11.2%), and the following with at least 20,000 of the 2009 new legal residents: Arizona, Georgia, Maryland, Massachusetts, Pennsylvania, Virginia, and Washington. These same states also lead in having the most foreign-born. New York City and Los Angeles each had over 4 million foreign-born, and Miami, Chicago, Washington, DC, Houston, Dallas, and San Francisco each had 1–2 million foreign-born (Batalova and Lee, 2014).

Annual net immigration (new permanent legal residents per year) is at 1.1 million per year. Approximately 104,000 foreigners arrive each day in the United States, of whom the majority are tourists, students, or business persons. While on average only 3,100 per day have immigrant visas allowing them to settle and become citizens after 5 years, another 2,000 unauthorized foreigners either overstay their legal visas or enter without papers across the Mexico-US border (Martin and Midgeley, 2010).

If the annual immigration continues at this same level of 1 million per year with the same composition of origin countries, between 2010 and 2050 the Hispanic population, which includes the immigrants from Latin America and their descendants, will double from 15.8% to 27.8% in 2050, and the Asian population will increase from 4.4% to 6.1% in 2050. The Black population will increase very slightly, from 12.9% to 13.2%. The non-Hispanic White population is expected to decline during this same period, from 67.0% to 57.8% (Ortman and Guarneri, 2010).

Who Are the Immigrants Coming to the United States?

In 2012, 1.03 million immigrants obtained legal residence in the United States. Over one third (41.6%) came for Asia, another third (31.8%) came from North America, 10.4% from Africa, and the balance from Europe, Oceania, and South America. Less than half (45.3%) of the new legal residents admitted in 2009 were male, but these gender differences even out over time (US Department of Homeland Security, 2013). As shown in Table 1.1, when the recent arrivals are merged with those here for all durations, the US-born and foreign-born both have balanced gender distributions. Among both recent immigrants and those here for all durations, half were in the prime working ages of 20–44 years (53.4% among recent immigrants, 51.9% 18–44 years old among all foreign-born), substantially higher than the 34.9% who are 18–44 years old among the US-born. In contrast, fewer recent immigrants were 45–64 years of age (18.1%) or 65 and over (5.2%), compared to the US-born (see later discussion). Among all foreign-born, however, the proportions 45 and older (40.4%) were similar to the proportion among the US-born (38.4%).

The most striking difference between the US-born and foreign-born is in their racial and ethnic composition. While the US-born are dominated by White, non-Hispanic persons (69.4%), the foreign-born are dominated by Hispanic (46.2%) and Asian and Pacific Islander (25.6%) persons. The US-born had somewhat more Black or African American than the foreign-born (13.2% vs. 8.5%), but these differences may be offset by the unequal proportions of "some other race" among the US-born and foreign-born, as the "some other race" may include mixtures of Black with other races or ethnicities not specified in these few categories.

Immigrants also differ from the US-born in sociodemographic characteristics. More adult immigrants are currently married than among the US-born: 58.6% versus 46.1%. Three times as many adult immigrants never completed high school, 30.8% compared to 10.32% among the US-born. More adult immigrants are in the labor force, and they are less likely to be unemployed than the US-born, 8.5% versus 9.5%. Yet, immigrant households are

Table 1.1 Selected Characteristics of the US Population by Nativity Status, American Community Survey 2012 (1-year estimates)

Characteristic	US-born	Foreign-born
	N = 273,089,382	N = 40,824,658
SEX AND AGE		
Male	49.3%	48.7%
Age		
Under 18 years	26.0%	6.3%
18–44 years	34.6%	48.8%
45–64 years	25.6%	31.4%
65+ years	13.8%	13.4%
Median age (years)	35.9	42.6
RACE AND HISPANIC OR LATINO ORIGIN		
White alone, not Hispanic or Latino	69.4%	18.7%
Black or African American	13.2%	8.5%
Asian and Pacific Islander	2.1%	25.6%
Some other race	3.1%	15.0%
Hispanic or Latino origin (of any race)	12.5%	46.2%
CHARACTERISTICS FOR PERSONS 16+ YEARS		
Currently married	46.1%	58.6%
Less than high school graduate (25 + year olds)	10.2%	30.8%
In labor force	62.8%	66.7%
Unemployed (% civilian labor force 16 + years)	9.5%	8.5%
POVERTY RATES (Previous 12 months)		
All households (200% poverty level)	33.8%	43.7%
Married-couple family with children <5 years (100% poverty level)	5.8%	12.5%
Female householder with children <5 years (100% poverty level)	48.3%	45.6%

(continued)

Table 1.1 Continued

Characteristic	US-born	Foreign-born
	N = 273,089,382	N = 40,824,658
HOUSING CHARACTERISTICS		
Renter-occupied housing units	34.0%	49.0%
Linguistically isolated households (no one with English less than "very well")	0.7%	27.6%

Source: American Community Survey 2012, Table S0501: Selected Characteristics of 2008–2012 American Community Survey, 1-Year Estimates (2012).

more likely to live in poverty, with 43.7% having incomes at or below 200% of poverty level, compared to only 33.8% of US-born households. Among families with children under age 5, the poverty rates are higher among married immigrant families (12.5%) than among comparable US-born families (5.8%). For female-headed households with children under 5, poverty rates are higher for the US-born than for the immigrant household.

There is some evidence of the usual custom among migrants to "double-up" and share housing with others, generally fellow migrants. While only one-third of the US-born households are renters, almost half of the immigrant households are renters. Finally, over one fourth of the immigrant households are linguistically isolated (27.6% versus 0.7%), having no adult member who is fluent in English.

Many more of the immigrant families are working poor. They may be working at jobs that offer little security in addition to lower pay, with both adults working one or two jobs just to pay rent and living expenses. The immigrants are also more likely to be disadvantaged by their minority status and subject to racism and other forms of discrimination aimed at minorities. Fewer have a basic high school education, and many are linguistically isolated and unable to communicate adequately with organizational representatives, let alone government officers, about their needs or situation. As will be discussed, these socioeconomic vulnerabilities have an impact on immigrant interactions with the health system and their overall ability to stay healthy.

Among the immigrant working poor, those who appear to be most vulnerable to economic uncertainty and social exclusion are the undocumented immigrants. According to a report from the Pew Hispanic Center (Passel and

Cohn, 2009), in 2008 there were an estimated 11.9 million unauthorized or undocumented immigrants in the United States, of whom 8.3 million are in the US labor force. Three fourths of the unauthorized are Hispanic, and most of these are Mexicans, primarily living in California, Texas, Florida, and New York, which together account for 51% of all the undocumented. In Nevada, California, Arizona, and New Jersey, about one in ten workers in the state are undocumented immigrants. Undocumented immigrants are less educated than US-born or legal immigrants. Together with the difficulties they have in obtaining work due to their immigrant status, their low educational attainment also consigns most to very low-status, low-security work, often as day laborers or other casual workers in farming, construction, janitorial or landscaping work, food services, production, or transportation. Not surprisingly, their median household income of $36,000 is well below the median of $50,000 for US-born workers. As long as they have an unauthorized status, many immigrants have little chance of attaining upward economic mobility and a comfortable life. When one thinks of a hand-to-mouth existence, this accurately describes the life for untold numbers of undocumented immigrants.

Yet they do dream, and they are more likely than the legal immigrants or the US-born to establish stable relationships and build families. Compared to the US-born and legal immigrants, many more (47%) of the unauthorized immigrants are couples with children, and 73% of their children are US citizens by birth. In 2008, there were over two times as many US-born than unauthorized immigrant children living in families in which at least one parent is unauthorized. Because of the low incomes of their parents, children of unauthorized immigrants are twice as likely to live in poverty, compared to children of US-born parents. The nature of their employment situation means that the unauthorized are much less likely to work in jobs that provide employer-sponsored health insurance plans, and even if they do, these plans are prohibitively expensive for immigrant families. Over half (59%) of the unauthorized immigrants have no insurance for themselves, and their children are also likely to go without health insurance—that is, 45% of the unauthorized immigrant children and 25% of the US-born children with unauthorized parents. Compared to children with legal immigrant or US-born parents, children of undocumented parents are most likely to go without any health insurance.

Compared to authorized or legal immigrants, unauthorized immigrants are likely to be more disadvantaged when it comes to investing in health, apart from the lack of insurance. Their employment situations may be more precarious, where taking time off from work to go to the doctor means risking the loss of one's job. They have less disposable income, and studies show that they in fact spend half or less on health care, compared to US-born men and women. When they do seek health care, they are more likely to have a negative experience due to language barriers, low health literacy, and underlying fears of interacting with "the system." While the Affordable Care Act aims to reduce insurance rates, undocumented immigrants were specifically excluded; they were not even allowed to purchase health insurance on the exchanges with their own money. Together these factors conspire against routine health care, leaving families to wait until the condition becomes urgent before seeking health care at the emergency department. Thus, they make fewer visits for health care, but when they do, they are sicker than US-born children brought to the emergency department (Gusmano, 2012).

Immigrants Recount Their Experiences

While the statistics clearly indicate that the experience of immigrating to the United States is a challenging one, it is difficult to appreciate how these challenges come together to influence how immigrants respond to the challenges they face. In the interviews we conducted with immigrants in 2011–2012, we asked them to recount their experiences upon arrival in the United States and how they addressed them. What we learned was that their situations upon arrival tended to be very precarious, living with others, having no source of income, and struggling against linguistic and cultural barriers to build a life. Job by job, month by month, they often faced discrimination and exploitation because of the vulnerability of their immigrant status. In this section of the chapter, we share the stories of immigrants we interviewed who we believe typify the struggles immigrants face and how this may shape their ability to address health concerns.

Arelia is a Peruvian immigrant, who came to the United States in 1993 at the age of 17 with her family. Her story illuminates the different strategies used by immigrants to establish themselves and build their lives: a long and arduous trip fleeing persecution to get to the United States, being hosted by a relative upon arrival, struggling to learn English and coping with situations where her English was inadequate, finding a job as an undocumented immigrant, discrimination and sexual exploitation by unscrupulous bosses, marriage to an American, night studies, and the gradual progression to establish herself in a stable job and career path.

In 1993, I was at school when the Shining Path terrorists attacked my school. I only survived because I was in the latrine at the time they attacked the school. My family found me there hours later, and my parents decided right then that we had to leave the country. I was 17 at the time, and my parents feared that the terrorists would come after me. Already, my father had lost his job of 28 years due to privatizing. In Peru, if you become unemployed after you are 30 years old, you can forget about finding another job. So, we knew he had no future there, so we all left. My uncle was already in the United States, and we decided to join him. While my uncle petitioned for us to come, my parents sold everything and we bought passage on a ship bound for the United States. So we left (my father, mother, my 13-year-old sister, and I). But it didn't turn out the way we expected. The ship stopped in Panama and abandoned us there. We were determined to go on, and besides we had no choice. We could not go back. So we walked, all the way through Mexico and up to California. It took 3 months to get to the United States. My uncle picked us up and we came to Sunnyside, Queens in New York City, where we, all of us, lived with my uncle. I still live here in Sunnyside.

Well, it was my dream to get a job and work in corporate America, speaking English (which I needed to learn). But once I arrived, people treated me like I was stupid because I didn't speak English. They treated me like I was alien, illegal, and it made me very sad. It was very hard to find my first job. Finally, I got a job in a factory, working 15 hours per day. I worked there without papers. I gave them a made-up social security number which I had invented. With my first check I bought clothes for everyone in my family, because it was winter, very cold, and we needed coats and boots. I worked there for a year. I met an American, fell in love, and we got married. At that time, if you married an American or someone with papers, you could get a permit to work after 3 months of marriage. So, I eventually got a permit to work, and then I found a job at a restaurant. I started as a waitress. I still didn't speak English, but I had learned the menu by memory, and I knew the words for the items on the menu. If customers wanted something different and used the word "instead," I did not understand, so I had to go to the kitchen to "check if it was OK," and then find out what the person requested in English from the kitchen staff, who translated the English "instead" words back into Spanish. Then, I would go back to the customer and confirm the order in English, using the words they had told me. So, I gave good service, I knew what they wanted.

All the while, I was working on learning English. I went on Saturdays to the library to learn English, and I was very happy. I went to Brooklyn Community College, and the teacher gave me permission to sit in, since I couldn't afford the fees. After a couple years, I did learn English. I was promoted from waitress to cashier at the restaurant. One Friday, I went in to the kitchen to chat about what we were going to do with our paychecks on this payday. To my surprise, the Mexican dishwashers said they were not being paid, because the owner said, "The restaurant did not have the money." But I knew they had the money in the cash register. So, I coached the Mexican dishwasher to ask for the money to pay the rent in the middle of the busy time, because he could not fire him during that busy time. But another person overheard me coaching the Mexican dishwashers to stand up for their rights, and he told the boss what he had heard, and I was fired. Of course, I got a job at another restaurant.

I had to renew my work permit every year. It took all day to wait for them to call me and then to renew it, and I had to pay $200 per year to be able to work for a year. I did this for 6 years, and gradually I was able to work my way up into a stable job with one of the health insurance companies, where I helped to enroll other families into the health plan. Then, after the sixth annual renewal, I got a letter saying that I had to go back to Peru because I had not renewed my permit. This was not true, but when I complained, they kept insisting. I was crying and crying and felt desperate. I went to my current boss, together we went to lawyers in New York City, and then to my congressional representative in Washington, DC. With her support plus the 35 letters of support I solicited to back up my residency application, after 3 months I finally got my residency.

The story of a 57-year-old Dominican immigrant working in a Head Start program goes into greater detail on the difficulties of finding work with the double burden of not knowing English and not having papers.

This is the country where you have the opportunity to be a professional if you want to or to be a delinquent if you want to. I spoke a little English when I joined my family in New York City. My mother and sister were working in a factory on 180th Street, and they found a job for me through their boss. I got my green card 1½ months after coming here. My job was at a dress factory where I worked on sections of the dress. I was at the factory for 2 years, then we moved to another factory downtown, where they gave us better pay.

I was there 6 months. Then I got another job at a factory producing soap and bleach in New Jersey, across the bridge from Washington Heights. I had to take the bus at 5:30 in the morning, and came home again at 5:00. I was there less than 6 months, because they changed the personnel every 3 months, so I was "let go." They don't want to do the paperwork to keep you there with your visa, so they fire you and then they hire new people.

Another immigrant who fled political persecution was Karime, who came from rural Mauritania, on the Senegal River. Unlike Arelia, however, he was able to establish his refugee status and obtained political asylum. While this did not solve all his living problems, his education and his status permitted him to advance and do things that it took much longer for Arelia to do. A life-long activist, Karime has continued to maintain a strong connection to his home region in Mauritania, going back each year for community and health development activities.

I am from Ka'edi, Mauritania, along the Senegal River. In 1986, the government upped the oppression against those of us along the Senegal River. Mauritanians had just been expelled by the Senegalese, and this became a rationale for the Mauritanian government to take action against us. Then, the oppression, killings, imprisonment, and human rights violations against our people got worse, each year, 1989 to 1992. Finally, in 1992 it became too dangerous for me when I was personally threatened. Already a few hundred people had been murdered by the government agents, so a group of us who were most threatened came to New York City. I applied for asylum when I came. The Mauritanian situation was well documented, and it was not difficult to build a case around that. I got help in preparing the application from organizations and their lawyers. It took about 2 years for the case to be settled. My case was actually very fast, as often it can take much longer. I was granted asylum, as did most of the other people who came with me.

I came to New York City, because New York City is the capital of human rights. You have the major human rights organizations here; it surpasses Thailand for activism. I thought I would be more effective by being here. Some people were already here from Ka'edi when I came, and I stayed with them when I first arrived. But most Mauritanians live in Ohio, where the living cost is low, and housing is accessible. Families can have their own space. And there are lots of jobs, good-paying jobs, compared to New York City. Plus, these jobs have medical coverage and benefits. The Mauritanians in

Ohio encourage others to come. News spreads very quickly. For those plan-ning to go to school, it is also easier to be in Ohio, because you can afford your own apartment while you go to school, and not have to share. Good-paying job, low rent—that brings the immigrants.

Immigrants from our home town, Ka'edi, have an association, and we all get together in Ohio once a year. We also help families back home. Each year we send a "health caravan" of doctors and health professionals who travel through our region for 7–10 days, providing health services to isolated com-munities along the river. We all contribute to this and it has been very suc-cessful. We also want to honor the communities where we visit, so we give awards to organizations or individuals who have contributed to the promo-tion of the language, culture, or well-being of the population. In this way we honor the entire community and create role models for others to strive for. Health Caravan has now become a nonprofit, dedicated to supporting health care for those in need, independent of government health services. Each year the organization supports bringing a child to the United States for surgery that cannot be done in Mauritania.

My dream really is to contribute to fundamental social change back home and in Africa, in general. I continue to be very focused on human rights and am in touch with people working on the human rights situation in Mauritania. In fact, I am in touch with many groups working for human rights in Africa. As emigrants, we are the driving energy to this effort. It is our vision and we have to make a contribution. I am also very active in Immigrant Rights Coalition here in New York.

People assign different missions to themselves. Whatever your mission, it is most important to have the courage to take risks in life. I have to believe that what is important is not your life, but what you can achieve in your life. So many people have sacrificed their lives in our country. Here, people also have sacrificed their lives, like Martin Luther King. He could have lived, but he took responsibility as a human being to make his contribution. That is what we all want to do. There are people who are part of history and there are people who make history. I don't want to be a part of history; I want to be a part of those who make history.

Karime's story reflects the courage, perseverance, and vision that drive immigrants to not only work hard for their own security but also for the community welfare. As will be discussed in later chapters, his energy and dedication to promoting social change are not unique and are part of the attributes that go into becoming a successful community health worker, which, by the way, Karime is. He, like others we have interviewed, overcame incredible odds and took huge risks to come to the United States. Immigrants often want to "give back" to other immigrants, to help them with their onward journeys.

More typical of the immigrant experience is the immigrant who joins a whole host of relatives who have come before, continuing along the pathways that have linked the United States with the homeland for perhaps decades. Maria's story is typical of an immigrant whose family and community connections before and after moving support her as she finds her way. In her case, this "wrap-around" community network may have slowed her in learning English, which ultimately has restricted her options, if not those of her children.

It was pretty much a given that I would come to New York, to the "Heights." I already had 20 relatives in the neighborhood. Back home, everyone knew the neighborhood where I ended up. We even knew the train and bus routes, the streets, everything, before we came.

Language has been far and away the biggest challenge. I failed the English proficiency exam, which prevents me from going to college and furthering my education. It's hard because I know lots of people back in the Dominican Republic who were able to go on and get better careers, like as a lawyer or a doctor, and I feel like I haven't accomplished as much. I really want a good and steady job, but my English skills have held me back. Even my daughters seem more Americano now, and they don't like to speak in Spanish, which leads to communication issues at home. I want a good job, but I am not very good at English. Which means I struggle to make ends meet. I would love to own my own house—to not have to pay the rent, which stresses me every month. I want my children to continue their studies and become successful professionals but also to retain their nationality and language.

Even for those lucky enough to have many family members upon whom to call for help, life is not easy, and each immigrant must make his or her own way. As they forge their own life, they are rightfully proud of what they are able to achieve, through sheer grit. Thus, when they are not able to do all that they dream of, it is discouraging to ask for help. They are embarrassed to seek public assistance, even though they know they are entitled to it, as the story of another Dominican immigrant reflects.

Before I came in 1982 I had a lot of family here. On my father's side, three uncles, two aunts, on my mother's side one aunt and a lot of cousins. They lived in Brooklyn, Washington Heights, and Queens. When I was 24, I came with a tourist visa. I only spoke Spanish. I first stayed with my uncle for a few months, in Brooklyn. My father had given me money to support me. I had done 2 years of college before coming, so then I enrolled in Boricua College to continue my studies. I moved to Washington Heights after only a few months when I married, but I continued with my studies. It was very hard at college, because my courses were in English. In 1984 I got my first job in a factory in New Jersey, making packaging for cosmetics. I stayed there for 11 months and then I went to another job which my cousin helped me to get, also in New Jersey, packaging medicines. I worked there for another 11 months, and then I said to myself, "This is not what I came to do in this country. I have to finish my college." So I quit and concentrated on my studies. In 1986 when my first child was born, I got welfare. I was very embarrassed to go there, because they treat people very bad and they made me feel very bad. Looking back, I feel very sad. I stayed on welfare from 1986 until I got this job in 1998. I finally graduated from Boricua in 1990. In 1996, I started at Harlem Hospital through the welfare-to-work program in the morning, and then I volunteered in the social work department. They helped me a lot, how to work with patients. In 1998 I was hired to work as a community health worker for the asthma program.

In addition to work, housing also poses challenges for immigrants, particularly those who do not have family to support them when they come, as is the case for many of the African immigrants we interviewed. An Ivoirian who came by himself when he could no longer tolerate being in his country's army talked about his first years. He had great resolve and was eventually able to get papers, an education, and a steady job.

I faced big challenges the first couple years. I didn't know anyone. I stayed one night with one person, and he then sent me to another place. Everyone was talking, talking, talking until 2 a.m. in the morning, and I couldn't sleep. It was in the Bronx. I was in a building where there were other Ivoirian and Guinean migrants, some who came straight from the village. We each had our own room, three floors were African and the other floors were mixed with immigrants from other countries. The total was around 50 Africans in this building alone. I was in that building for 3 years and then I realized I had to move somewhere else to learn English.

It is very, very painful to come here as an immigrant without any papers. If you don't have citizenship or papers, it is hard to get education or a job. You have to be very strong. Not to be involved with drugs and alcohol to help you forget. But I came here for something else. I could have done alcohol and drugs, but that was not what I came for. I came to make a better life. It is hard when you first come, when you realize that it is not easy and see the whole picture about how you have to struggle to work outside—wash the store windows, sweep, be on the street, work more than 24 hours. You have to make sure that you pay your taxes, as this will help you to become a part of it and do what you want to do.

Every day when I wake up it is a blessing when I see where I am now, and this keeps me going. My mom, her strength, is keeping me going and my dreams speak to her. She never gave up. She stayed because of us, and that gives me strength. My brother and sister came to thank me, and that helped me, too. When you finally get papers and education, then this is a country of opportunity and you have to grab it. I love this country. I am blessed.

Immigrants and Health: The Issues

Immigrants are focused on establishing themselves, finding a job, and creating a home and family in their new residence. Many maintain strong connections to their home by sending money home and when possible making return visits to the family back home. Even those forced out by economic, political, or environmental crises find themselves joining voluntary migrants in pursuing opportunities to settle and build a new life. Health is usually not the first concern of immigrants, and like their nonimmigrant counterparts, health does not become an issue until it is forced upon the immigrant as the experience of disease, disability, or, in the case of women, pregnancy and childbirth. The interactive process by which immigrants generate a livelihood and health is shown in Figure 1.1. This model shows that immigrants combine a host of community resources with their own resources to pursue alternative livelihood and health options. Their own human and social capital will play a key role in pursuing opportunities, although assets and savings can enable them to invest in additional education in order to move up the professional career ladder. If they are able to have all the resources they need, they can gain the prize of sustainable livelihoods and health.

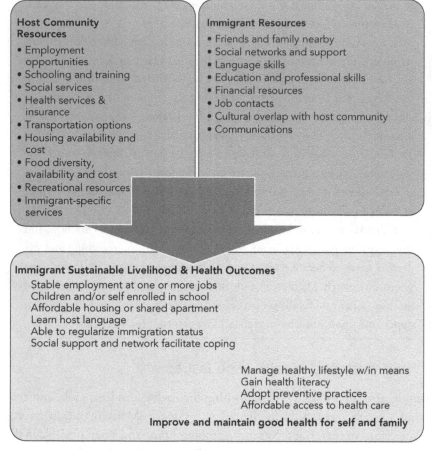

Host Community Resources

- Employment opportunities
- Schooling and training
- Social services
- Health services & insurance
- Transportation options
- Housing availability and cost
- Food diversity, availability and cost
- Recreational resources
- Immigrant-specific services

Immigrant Resources

- Friends and family nearby
- Social networks and support
- Language skills
- Education and professional skills
- Financial resources
- Job contacts
- Cultural overlap with host community
- Communications

Immigrant Sustainable Livelihood & Health Outcomes

Stable employment at one or more jobs
Children and/or self enrolled in school
Affordable housing or shared apartment
Learn host language
Able to regularize immigration status
Social support and network facilitate coping

Manage healthy lifestyle w/in means
Gain health literacy
Adopt preventive practices
Affordable access to health care

Improve and maintain good health for self and family

FIGURE 1.1 Interactive Processes Affecting Immigrant Sustainable Livelihoods and Health Outcomes

Most immigrants have time on their side in terms of overall health risks. Because immigrants cluster in the prime working age years, many benefit from a long postimmigration period when their risks of ill health and disease are at their lowest. This makes it easier to maintain good health without costly investments in terms of money, time, or information seeking. In addition, immigrants are more likely to be of somewhat higher educational or economic status, both because they have the resources to immigrate and because they seek the kinds of educational and economic opportunities not available in their home countries (Gushulak and Macpherson, 2006). Whether through their youth or educational and economic status, immigrants tend to be healthier than those who do not migrate in their home country, and they are also likely to be in better health than comparable native-born people.

This positive selectivity for good health is known as the "healthy migrant" effect, and it has been well documented, particularly among Latinos, specifically Mexican Americans, coming to the United States (Abraido-Lanza, Dohrenwend, Ng-Mak, and Turner, 1999; Jasso, Massey, Rosenzweig, and Smith, 2004; Martin and Midgeley, 2010).

The healthy migrant effect is evident in the overall mortality patterns as well as in specific disease risk. In the United States in 2003, immigrant life expectancy was 80.0 years, as compared to 76.6 for US-born. The Asian and Pacific Islander immigrants had the highest life expectancies, while the lowest were found among Black immigrants, who were about the same as US-born Blacks, with Hispanics in between. In 2003, immigrants had 30% or more lower mortality for lung and esophageal cancer, chronic obstructive pulmonary disease, suicide, and HIV/AIDS but 50% or more higher mortality for stomach and liver cancer (Singh and Hiatt, 2006). A more recent analysis of death rates among persons aged 25 and above by age, gender, race/ethnicity, and nativity showed that lower death rates found among Hispanics were only found among Hispanic women, and more specifically only those who were not of Mexican origin. Foreign-born non-Hispanic Blacks had lower death rates than their US-born counterparts (Borrell and Lancet, 2012).

Because the US benefit programs specifically target women and young children, immigrant women and their preschool children have access to reproductive health services and nutritional support programs, enabling healthier pregnancies, deliveries, and infants. Women born in Sub-Saharan Africa appear to benefit from these services more than Caribbean immigrants, as their rates of preterm delivery or small-for-gestational-age infants is lower than for the Caribbean-born, but both have more favorable birth outcomes than African Americans (Elo, Vang, and Culhane, 2014). There is evidence that Mexican immigrants also take advantage of these services, as they have better birth outcomes and children with lower infant mortality rates than US-born women (Guendelman, Thornton, Gould, and Hosang, 2006; Hummer, Powers, Pullum, Gossman, and Frisbie, 2007; Wingate and Alexander, 2006). The healthy migrant effect may or may not be continued as the children grow, as there is some evidence from the United States that children of immigrant families use health care services less and are in worse physical health than children in nonimmigrant families (Guendelman, Angulo, Wier, and Oman, 2005; Guendelman, Schauffler, and Pearl 2001). While first-generation or foreign-born children were 26% less likely to be obese than native-born children, differences emerged for second-generation children, among whom the Hispanic children were more likely while the

Asian children were less likely than US-born Whites to be overweight (Singh, Kogan, and Yu, 2009). National survey data show that 23% of immigrant Hispanic children are physically inactive, compared to 9.5% of US-born White children with US-born parents, and they are half as likely to participate in sports (Singh, Yu, Siahpush, and Kogan, 2008).

If the immigrants have traditions of protective health behaviors, such as avoiding alcohol or tobacco, when these traditions are maintained, the healthy migrant effect can continue after their arrival as they continue to practice these protective behaviors (Akresh and Frank, 2008; Jasso et al., 2004; Wingate and Alexander, 2006). After controlling for socioeconomic status, gender, race, and age, immigrants were less likely to smoke cigarettes, to be overweight or obese, to have activity limitations, or to perceive themselves to be in poor health (Singh and Hiatt, 2006). Within comparable race or ethnicity groups, immigrants generally had better health outcomes for almost all major disease categories (Argeseanu Cunningham, Ruben, and Narayan 2008).

As shown in Figure 1.1, when immigration enables families to move out of poverty, they are able to invest in quality of life improvements that support better health, such as improved diet and access to health care, paid for out of pocket or through insurance through employment (Adler and Ostrove, 1999). Immigrants with higher educational attainment generally contribute to the observed lower mortality and better health among immigrants (Singh and Siahpush, 2002). However, those with lower educational attainment and those working at low-skill occupations have poorer health outcomes, which is linked to financial stress, which is in turn linked to more smoking, more sedentary behavior, and greater obesity risk (Siahpush, Heller, and Singh, 2005; Siahpush et al., 2014).

Just as immigrants get help from other fellow immigrants in finding jobs and housing, fellow immigrants can also point the way to services needed to improve health. Adapting to a new living situation can be stressful, and the social support that immigrants receive from others in the community reduces that stress. Through their social networks, immigrants can receive valuable information about health care services, as well as emotional support, both of which contribute to better health and reduced mortality (Berkman and Syme, 1979; Loucks et al., 2006). When immigrants are able to interact with others, they become integrated into the community, which has proven a successful strategy for promoting both livelihoods and health. Immigrants who have overcome institutional barriers to obtaining health care have often cited information and support from friends and family as one of the pathways to their success (Litwin,

2010; Salinero-Fort et al., 2011). Such information and the social support to use it can contribute to closing the gap between how immigrants traditionally view their health problems and the prevention or treatments recommended by the health care system (Edberg, Cleary, and Vyas, 2010).

In reality, the economic and survival needs of the immigrant often trump health concerns, and the secondary outcomes of health depicted in Figure 1.1 are not achieved. Health is not a "free" good, and immigrants struggling to survive or to get ahead may not be able to sustain the financial or time investments needed to stay healthy, such as food, insurance, medications, information and coaching, time for social support and networking, and time for preventive behaviors (Derose, Escarce, and Lurie 2007; Edberg et al., 2010).

About half of all immigrants to the United States do not have health insurance, either because they work at low-wage jobs where health insurance is not offered by the employer or they cannot afford the insurance premiums (Capps, Rosenblum, and Fix 2009). Recent immigrants are not eligible for health insurance, and even if they or their children are eligible, mistrust of the government or the health care system may keep them from applying for this insurance. If they are undocumented immigrants, fear of being reported can prevent immigrants from accessing public assistance for eligible children. In addition, those in the country on a family reunification visa are unable or unwilling to use publicly funded health care services, which could imply that their sponsor is not covering their expenses. Others planning to bring others in on a family reunification visa are loath to have any record of depending on governmental subsidies or services, including for health care (Stewart et al., 2006). Thus, US-born children of immigrants are less likely to have health insurance than are children of US-born parents (Capps and Fix, 2013). Those without the requisite language or educational skills may end up in part-time or shift work where simply going to the doctor may require taking off work and loss of income. Simply going to the doctor is prohibitively expensive for them. Thus, immigrants will put off going to the doctor until their symptoms become so acute they cannot ignore them (Hagan, Rodriguez, Capps, and Kabiri, 2003; Pati and Danagoulian, 2008).

Prevention or timely treatment is a luxury for the uninsured immigrant. The lack of preventive or routine care increases the chance that the early signs of illness will be missed, and treatment may only be sought when the condition reaches an advanced stage requiring intensive and often costly intervention (Gushulak and Macpherson, 2006; Lasser, Himmelstein, and Woolhandler, 2006; Lassetter and Callister, 2009; Uiters, Deville, Foets, Spreeuwenberg, and Groenewegen, 2009).

Further, more income does not necessarily translate into better health. While in general more education and higher income are associated with fewer medical conditions or functional impairments, this varies greatly by immigrant group. There appears to be a weaker link between socioeconomic status and health among Mexican immigrants (Acevedo-Garcia, Soobader, and Berkman, 2007; Goldman, Kimbro, Turra, and Pebley, 2006). Among Puerto Ricans (who are natural-born US citizens) the positive status effect on health operates through income, among Cubans socioeconomic status has marginal effects, and among Mexicans the socioeconomic effects are reversed, with poorer health among higher status Mexicans than among lower status Mexicans (Zsembik and Fennell, 2005). The impact of education on reducing smoking and obesity is different for men and women and for Mexicans by duration of residence. Education has little effect on smoking prevalence among men and women born in Mexico, regardless of duration living in the United States, while it does have an effect among US-born Whites and, to a lesser extent, US-born Mexicans. Education also has little relation to obesity among different groups of male Mexican immigrants, but among women there are strong education-obesity relations, with an inverse relation among all women except among recent arrivals, for whom education above high school is associated with higher obesity (Buttenheim, Goldman, Pebley, Wong, and Chung, 2010).

The variation in the association between socioeconomic status and health behaviors or outcomes among immigrants may reflect the different ways that living in the United States affects health. While immigrants may arrive with a higher health status, associated with their age or educational status, this health status is expected to converge toward the pattern found in their host community. While the concept of "acculturation" remains problematic in its potentially homogeneous views of origin and host "cultures," acculturation attempts to address the process by which immigrant values and behavioral norms become a blend of the "old," those originating in their homeland, and the "new," those evident in the host neighborhood or community, even if not at a national level in either location (Lara, Gamboa, Kahramanian, Morales, and Bautista, 2005; Siatkowski, 2007). When immigrants do not speak English, for example, they may remain unfamiliar with the health care system and therefore not know how to seek care when they do fall ill (Cordasco, Ponce, Gatchell, Traudt, and Escarce, 2011; Sable, Campbell, Schwarz, Brandt, and Dannerbeck, 2006). When immigrants interact primarily with other immigrants, they may continue to be strongly influenced by the views of health and illness common to people at their origin (Caban and Walker, 2006).

Traditional values may be particularly important in shaping the symbolic and social meaning of food. Among some immigrant groups, eating large quantities of high-fat or high-protein foods is considered a sign of status (Finucane and McMullen, 2008; Renzaho, Gibbons, Swinburn, Jolley, and Burns, 2006). Efforts to change nutritional habits among immigrants often have been slow to produce change, due to the mixed messages of the new and old cultures. Compared to US-born Whites, Latinos have had more difficulty in adopting healthy diet recommendations, partly because it is difficult for them to find and buy recommended foods but also because of a desire to adopt the popular American fast-food culture (Horowitz, Colson, Hebert, and Lancaster, 2004; Horowitz, Tuzzio, Rojas, Motheith, and Sisk, 2004; Perez-Escamilla, 2011). As a result, with longer residence in the United States they are more likely to be obese and have cardiovascular diseases (Kaushal, 2009; Mainous, Diaz, and Geesey, 2008; Wolin, Colangelo, Chiu, and Gapstur, 2009).

The stress of seeking work and establishing a family in an unfamiliar community is often detrimental to health, particularly health outcomes associated with healthy lifestyles, such as hypertension (Gadd, Sundquist, Johansson, and Wandell, 2005; Gushulak and Macpherson, 2006). Immigrants may take up smoking, which is linked to much higher cardiovascular and pulmonary disease. Others may turn to alcohol or other substances that are part of the culture and living situation in which they find themselves (Antecol and Bedard, 2006; Lara et al., 2005; Stoddard, 2009). Recent evidence also shows that immigrants are being swept into the obesity epidemic, with higher than average overweight and obesity rates (Kaushal, 2009; Singh et al., 2009).

Because immigrants are more likely to be poor and to be in rental housing, they tend to reside in low-income neighborhoods, which are also less likely to have the kinds of services and facilities necessary to support healthy lifestyles, such as safe sidewalks, parks, fitness centers, and jogging paths (Edberg et al., 2010; Stoddard, 2009). Whether because of their living situations or their occupations, immigrants also may have higher than average exposure to environmental toxins. In the San Joaquin Valley where many Mexican immigrants live and work, families in the poorest communities had more low birth weight infants, childhood asthma hospitalizations, and disability days than those in the less vulnerable communities (Huang and

London, 2012). Higher exposure to environmental toxins in the poorer communities also can increase the risk of cancer or other noncommunicable diseases (Gushulak and Macpherson, 2006; Macintyre et al., 2003). Such environmental exposures among Asian and Pacific Islander immigrants may contribute to their poorer mental health, cardiovascular health, cancer outcomes, injuries and overall mortality than US-born of the same ethnicity. Poor living conditions and crowding may also contribute to the higher rates of diabetes and infectious disease outcomes among Hispanics (Argeseanu Cunningham et al., 2008).

Overlaying this complex set of social, economic, cultural, and environmental vulnerabilities affecting immigrant health are the discriminatory processes built into so many layers of US society. As Krieger and colleagues have shown in their work, racial discrimination against Blacks applies to both immigrant and US-born Blacks. In addition to their higher rates of poverty, both groups of Blacks encounter frequent episodes of discrimination, resulting in a seven-fold increase in their severe psychological health (Krieger, Kosheleva, Waterman, Chen, and Koenen, 2011). Discrimination is also evident for Latinos. While recent immigrants and first-generation Latinos may not perceive this as strongly, attributing the attitudes to their immigrant status rather than to their ethnicity or background, the second generation appears to be more likely to perceive their social exclusion from mainstream society, a process described as "othering" and observed among Mexican immigrants in Michigan (Viruell-Fuentes, 2007). Discrimination and stress have also been observed among Dominican immigrant women in New York City (Panchanadeswaran and Dawson, 2011) and among Latino immigrant men in North Carolina (Ornelas, Eng, and Perreira, 2011) and in Oregon (McClure et al., 2010). Among immigrant men, especially young men and the second generation of immigrant youth, the combined experiences of poverty and discrimination increase the chances of binge drinking and substance abuse (Edberg et al., 2010; Ornelas et al., 2011). Thus, the multiple oppressions of poverty, community disadvantage, and discrimination may be the underlying forces behind the observed rise in alcohol abuse and smoking among immigrants with longer durations of residence in the United States (Abraido-Lanza, Chao, and Florez, 2005; Finch and Vega, 2003; Romero, Martinez, and Carvajal, 2007; Viruell-Fuentes, 2007). When there is a high degree of social network homogeneity among groups who share daily discrimination, this further reinforces the patterns of behaviors, such as substance abuse or smoking, associated with attempts to find alternative sources of self-esteem and control (Rostila, 2010; Viruell-Fuentes, Miranda, and Abdulrahim, 2012). Although immigrant networks can have a protective effect against covert discrimination in public or work settings (Torres, Yznaga, and Moore, 2011), there is no guarantee for this buffering effect.

While immigrants face the same health risks that others face, they must do so with fewer resources and greater vulnerability than the native born of similar economic status. They may not differ in the incidence of different health conditions, but they are much constrained in how they cope with them. Thus, immigrants, particularly the low-income immigrants who have no or inadequate insurance, cannot simply go to a doctor for treatment. Of overriding importance are the issues of access to health insurance and to health care providers who they can trust and interact with, but a more basic issue is the reactive pattern of interactions with the health care system, only "fixing what is broken," namely when symptoms become so great they cannot be ignored. To address specific health problem areas such as diabetes or cardiovascular disease will require a shift to proactive interactions with the health care system to manage illness before it becomes critical. To address the serious issues of diabetes and cardiovascular illness or other chronic conditions such as obesity or depression, different approaches are needed that will engage immigrants in their communities and enable them to learn about and embrace changes to their lifestyle and health-related behaviors. The problems of access to care, trust of the provider, and ability to take a proactive, preventive stance are interrelated, and the solutions likewise need to be integrated.

Immigrant Experiences With Health Issues

As the immigrant stories show, there is little room in immigrants' lives to be sick or to invest much time or energy in staying healthy. Consistent with the statistics reported earlier in the chapter, they often do not have health insurance, and are often quite unfamiliar with how insurance works in the United States. When asked about how they dealt with health issues, virtually all those interviewed reported dealing with health problems only when they became urgent and could not be ignored. For women, the experience of pregnancy without health insurance was an eye opener, but also better than for other emergent concerns, since pregnant women and infants up to age 1 year are generally covered through Medicaid or specialized state insurance plans.

A Bangladeshi man, Abdul, described the challenges he and others in his community faced simply in going to the doctor, taking time off and then not knowing what to do or who to see when they do get to the doctor.

> When I came over here, I needed to get some health services, and I didn't know where to go, and I could not get help from anyone. My father has diabetes, and I had to help him. At Bellevue Hospital, people cannot communicate with the doctor. Language is a barrier. I had to help make appointments, remind about them, help him explain to the doctor. I see what happens to other immigrants. People cannot make the time to go to doctors. Sometimes they miss appointments. Hard to schedule, especially when their work schedules are so intense. They are just not able to come. They have to work, or they have child care responsibilities.

Several of the immigrants we spoke with recounted the well-documented pattern of ignoring health problems until they became so urgent that they had to go to the emergency room. Arelia's story continues, as she explains how her family was dependent on the emergency room for care.

> All this time I was paying taxes, Medicaid and social security, and we never got anything free from this country. No one in my family had checkups or physicals during that time. I didn't have a checkup until I was 22, and luckily I was very healthy. For ten years we did not go to the doctor for checkups, and even then we had terrible doctors who just looked in our eyes and didn't really check us. We used emergency room as primary care, because the ER did not ask for papers. We had to pretend to have a very bad headache or stomach ache to be seen. All these tricks we had to learn to be seen. We did have to go into the payment plans for the hospital, but I asked friendly people for help so they told us what to do.

Not all immigrants were as fortunate as Arelia and her family. Marielena from Panama described the difficulties she faced in getting her asthma under control.

> I must have had asthma all my life, because I had all those symptoms. But no one ever told me. Before I got diagnosed, I would do home remedies,

like honey and lemon, Vicks on the chest, and rest—it was "fatigue" in Panama. I would first tell myself that I would get better, take some tea, and it will get better. After I got a dog, it didn't get better so I went to the ER and they told me I had asthma. But the doctor didn't explain very much about what it was. I was afraid because I thought I was going to die and not be able to fulfill my dreams. I didn't have any insurance or benefits. So, I didn't know what to do. When I got sick and had symptoms, I was scared to use my name at the hospital. Finally, when I went to the hospital, I discovered that even if I didn't have insurance they would take care of me. By this time, my papers were coming through so then I could get insurance.

Even when the immigrant's health insurance is covered, interactions with the health care system may still be immensely challenging for immigrants who do not speak the language of the provider and are unfamiliar with the US health care system. We interviewed a young Colombian woman in Chicago about the challenges she faced during a visit when she developed complications with her pregnancy.

I came here to visit my family. My mom, my sister, and my cousin live here in the United States. I was pregnant and started having problems. I knew I needed health care. Helped by a friend who went through the same experience as a pregnant immigrant, I went to a nearby health clinic. The doctors told me that I had a high-risk pregnancy. Under the circumstances, I could not wait to go back to my country, so I was obliged to stay in the United States while expecting my baby. I was told that I needed to go to a bigger hospital due to my high-risk pregnancy. Again, my only help came from my family's friend. Otherwise, I would have been totally lost, because it was a big university hospital where most of the people do not speak Spanish.

I always felt unsure of myself. Nobody offered me any help in understanding or navigating the system. The only thing that was helpful for me was that in the majority of the doctor's visits I had a translator, but during the lab test or during the test to monitor the pregnancy I did not have a translator and I could not understand anything or ask questions. I did not know how I was, how my baby was. I felt impotent, unsecure. One day I had a sonogram that came out unsatisfactory. I barely understood that something was wrong with my baby, because I could not ask or say anything. They did not offer me translation. So, I went home and waited for eight days to the next doctor's visit to know what was happening. That was a time of anguish for me.

> The most helpful resources I had were my family's friend, the one I mentioned before, and one social worker that I met at the beginning of this process and who helped me some to apply for health care services. If they were not there, I cannot even think what I would have done. Unfortunately, they helped me only at the beginning. Most of the time I was dealing alone with the hospital system. During many of my doctor's visits as well as lab tests I was by myself trying to understand the health system alone.

Problems understanding the health care system and how it works are not limited to the undocumented immigrants. A young Polish immigrant in San Diego described the shock he had when he discovered that the US health care system was "pay as you go," whether by the patient or by his insurance.

> Well, I mean, the whole system was kind of hard for us to figure out because we both come from countries where we had a public health system. They take money from our taxes, which are higher than they are here, and we don't pay for anything when we have to go to see the physician, other than the private one, which is an option but you don't have to take it. So for us, it was difficult to figure out how the insurance worked, and I was surprised that people are not always sure what the prices are. Now, we kind of know how it works, and we have general physicians and pediatricians, but it is still hard to figure out how the insurance works. At least, we know where we need to go when we need any help.

These reflections from the immigrants we interviewed put a human side to the statistics portraying the difficulties and barriers encountered by immigrants in staying healthy. Behind the statistics are real families who have to juggle the many competing demands in their lives to deal with health problems, time and again relying on friends and family to help them speak with the doctor and learn what they have to do. For most, there is not one single problem that can be fixed, such as by a telephone interpretation service. It is not just the translation of the names of medications and how to take them that the immigrants need. It is also translation of what diseases like asthma or diabetes are, the whole concept that they can be managed or prevented, something the Panamanian immigrant never understood from her doctor. Beyond this translation of concepts are all the system issues that challenge immigrants, knowing which doctors to go to, how to go to doctors when they are not urgently sick, how to deal with insurance. Friends and family can help for some of these issues, but these are precisely the problems that community health workers can also address, as we will see in the next chapter. When asked whether a community health worker might have been helpful to her family in dealing with her health issues, Anna, the Russian immigrant, shared her views:

> Now, we're so Americanized that we don't need that help. But I can certainly envision that in the first few years, when you don't know much about your new environment, that somebody like that could definitely be helpful, because the health system here can be pretty complex and pretty hard to navigate. New immigrants coming would definitely benefit from somebody who can explain what's going on in terms that they can understand. Nurses and doctors have very well-defined jobs that they have to do; it's all very business-like, boom boom boom, like "What are your symptoms? Are you sick? Okay," then moving on to the next patient.
>
> I would say especially as somebody with a long-term condition, like me, somebody who doesn't just need to see the doctor once but needs long-term medical care, they need to know more than just what pills to take. They need to know about insurance and payment and financial options. They need to know how to fill the prescriptions, how to maintain regimens, what else they have to do besides prescriptions, maybe dietary, maybe non-pill options they have. Doctors can certainly prescribe something or recommend something, but actually getting people to maintain a full regimen for whatever they need will require more than the occasional doctor's visit. Rather than see them in at a particular doctor's visit, I would say somebody whose job it is to make sure that somebody stays healthy would help.
>
> And then, of course, if they share the same cultural background and language, then that's helpful for someone who doesn't speak the language or know the culture. In our Russian community, people have preconceptions and certain things they believe about health care, that, in my opinion, aren't always true or are distorted. Some of it is cultural and some of it is just, you know, clinging to things they learned prior to immigrating to the United States. So, I think just having someone like a community health worker, who would bridge the gap between this kind of closed—not necessarily closed, but self-sustaining and self-enforcing community of opinions—and American health care, would potentially be very beneficial. I think that it's such a big, difficult, and important topic and people just have so many misconceptions about health care, that having somebody that you can rely on, who's culturally the same, can be a big help.

The millions of immigrants in the United States, particularly those most vulnerable who have no insurance and limited resources and who lack the linguistic and cultural backgrounds for making good use of the health care system, could benefit from the community health worker of Anna's dreams. In the next chapter we will see to what extent there is evidence for pursuing Anna's vision for improved health through community health workers bridging the gap between the immigrants and the American health care system.

2

A Good Fit: Community Health Workers and Immigrant Health

COMMUNITY HEALTH WORKERS (CHWs) have been around for decades, and they are found in communities throughout the world. There are millions of CHWs, with most in the Third World, working in small rural areas that have little or no access to health care (Bhutta, Lassi, Pariyo, and Huicho, 2010). There are few fixed attributes for who can be a CHW; they may be old or young, male or female. However, it is central that they are welcomed and accepted by the community as people who can help others deal with health problems. In rural communities throughout the Third World, they are the village health workers who go from village to village, gathering men and women together to talk about things they can do to protect themselves or their children from illnesses such as diarrhea or malaria; in the world's cities, they might be working in low-income neighborhoods helping at-risk individuals prevent or manage their diabetes. They are known by many different names, but the essence of CHWs is that they are trusted members of the community where they work, and they have been selected to serve as liaisons between the health system and the community. Some have little or no training and work primarily to mobilize and activate the population, while others may be trained to educate their fellow community residents on a variety of health topics, primarily preventive but in some cases curative. For most, this training is usually "just enough" to enable them to carry out specific activities, ranging from a few hours to a couple of months (Li, Goethals, and Dorfman, 2008; Tran, Portela, de Bernis, and Beek, 2014).

If they have such limited training, can they make a difference in helping people become healthy, Anna's dream of CHWs who "bridge the gap" for new immigrants? In this chapter we first will review the evidence that supports use of CHWs to promote health, particularly for chronic disease prevention and control. Such reviews have already been completed by others, so this will simply be an updating from the latest reviews, which date from 2010. The bulk of the chapter focuses on summarizing the evidence that CHWs have thus far been successful in promoting the health of immigrants to the United States, which goes straight to Anna's dream. There are no prior reviews of the evidence focusing on how CHWs promote the health of immigrants in the United States, so this review is more detailed. After reviewing the evidence, we can outline how CHWs have thus far been able to bridge the gap between immigrants and the health system, in support of Anna's dream.

Evidence for Community Health Workers Contributing to Improving Health

Three major CHW program reviews published in 2010 were positive about the impact of CHWs on health outcomes.

The 2010 review by the Global Health Workforce Alliance (GHWA), conducted by Bhutta and colleagues, used broadly inclusive criteria for their review, including quasi-experimental, pre/post and descriptive study designs (Bhutta et al., 2010). This allowed them to include 320 studies, many times more than are usually included in Cochrane reviews, and with the inclusion of less rigorous studies, more studies were included from moderate- and low-income settings ($n = 261$). In addition to assessing whether the studies provided sufficient evidence of a positive impact of CHWs on improving health outcomes pertaining to the Millennium Development Goals (MDGs), they also reviewed the evidence regarding the performance and functionality of the CHWs, including types of training (duration and content), supervision, incentives, and support received by the CHWs. With this broader perspective, they were able to include studies pertaining to a very diverse group of CHWs, including those with only a few days of training up to 2 years of training.

The GWHA review team found that CHWs provided a wide range of services contributing to the MDGs for nutrition, child health, maternal health, and adult health (malaria/TB/HIV noncommunicable diseases [NCDs]/mental health), and they recommended continued expansion of the CHW cadre. The strongest evidence for CHW contributions were for promotion of antenatal and postnatal care; promotion of early and exclusive breastfeeding; ensuring a safe delivery; reduction of newborn infections and neonatal mortality; home management of uncomplicated childhood illnesses (diarrhea, malaria, pneumonia) using ORT, zinc, and antibiotics supplied by the CHW; appropriate care seeking for childhood illnesses; promotion of childhood immunizations; preventive health education for malaria, HIV/AIDS, and other sexually transmitted diseases; prevention of chronic diseases; and counseling to address mental health problems (Bhutta et al., 2010). These are extraordinary findings. A subsequent distillation of 26 studies of CHW contributions to improving management of diarrhea and pneumonia showed that community case management by CHWs significantly improved appropriate management and use of ORT, zinc, and antibiotics, as well as more appropriate care seeking for sick children, leading to a reduction in mortality associated with diarrhea or pneumonia (Bhutta et al., 2013).

Based on the dozen program case studies conducted for programs in Africa and Asia, the GWHA study concluded that CHW impact on reducing newborn, infant, child, and maternal mortality could have been greater if the training had been more interactive, equipping the CHW with stronger health education skills and if they had more frequent and supportive supervision, preferably combined with refreshers. They identified the following factors limiting the range and quality of CHWs and their potential impact: shortage of commodities and drugs, inadequate and irregular supervision, lack of functional equipment, insufficient training, mentoring or refreshers, low status and low remuneration, and inadequate linkages to the health system (Bhutta et al., 2010). As will be seen in the succeeding chapters, many of these same operational issues are important to the success of CHW programs working with immigrants in the United States.

The two reviews that included studies conducted primarily in the United States or other high-income countries used more stringent standards for including studies and hence included a much smaller number; in fact, fewer than 100 met the requisite standards for study design of a Cochrane review. In their review of 53 studies on CHW interventions in the United States, Vishwanatham and colleagues applied a health behavior approach to assessing the impact of CHWs (Viswanathan et al., 2009). They found mixed evidence regarding CHW impact on participant knowledge or behavior change and health care utilization, along with mixed evidence regarding their impact on health outcomes. The specific health conditions for which there was evidence of CHW contributions to improved health outcomes were not dissimilar to those found by the GWHA study: childhood immunizations, prenatal care and perinatal outcomes, child development and well-being, diabetes management, and asthma management. In addition, there was evidence that CHWs increased appropriate utilization of health care services, with improved rates of follow-up visits for several conditions and reduced emergency department visits for asthma. The 2010 Cochrane review of 82 qualifying studies by Lewin and colleagues found similar findings for childhood immunizations, breastfeeding, and appropriate health care utilization (e.g., seeking care for sick children); the global studies included in the Lewin 2010 review also provided evidence that CHWs promote exclusive breastfeeding, improve TB treatment outcomes, and contribute to reducing neonatal mortality and child morbidity (Lewin et al., 2010).

These reviews all underscore the contribution of CHWs to changing maternal and child health care behaviors and outcomes, but to a lesser extent their impact on behaviors affecting adult health outcomes. In part, this reflects the depth of experimentation with CHWs for the last 40 years in the areas of maternal and child health, as part of nationally supported programs, such as Healthy Families or its variants, programs that include home visitation to support healthy pregnancy and parenting (Olds et al., 2002, 2004). Since the early 2000s, many more states and programs are experimenting with CHWs to help people prevent or manage chronic diseases, to adopt healthy lifestyles, to address issues of mental health that intersect with other chronic disease problems, and to support patient-centered medical homes. Therefore, it is particularly important to assess the effectiveness of CHWs for chronic disease prevention and management, as those pose significant threats for immigrants.

Diabetes Prevention

There was an explosion in studies reporting on the experience of incorporating CHWs into diabetes prevention and control programs, including an updated assessment of this experience by Shah and colleagues (Shah, Kaselitz, and Heisler, 2013). The more recent studies (published from 2009 forward) provide considerably more evidence concerning the effectiveness of CHWs to improve lifestyles that prevent diabetes (Babamoto et al., 2009; Baker, Simpson, Lloyd, Bauman, and Singh, 2011; Ockene et al., 2012; Ruggiero, Oros, and Choi, 2011). Many of these use adaptations of the CDC Diabetes Prevention Program, specifically the 16 sessions to promote lifestyle changes (Albright and Gregg, 2013). The adaptations that have been most successful were ones in which the lifestyle coaches, who include nurses, dieticians, social workers, certified health educators, or CHWs, were trained using interactive methodologies with small groups in which they could practice problem solving — as opposed to lecture presentations. In addition to this training, it is also important for the CHWs or lifestyle coaches to have a link to the health care system, as this promotes quality assurance and sustainability (Venditti and Kramer, 2013). Across the 28 adaptations of the DPP, CHWs were equally effective as health personnel in delivering the lifestyle program, with participants averaging 4% weight loss regardless of the type of personnel giving the program (Ali, Echouffo-Tcheugui, and Williamson, 2012). The most prominent adaptation of the DPP is delivery of the educational sessions at local YMCAs by CHWs trained to be lifestyle coaches, now at 46 different YMCAs (Ackerman, 2013; Ackerman, Finch, Brizendine, Zhou, and Marrero, 2008). Most (89%) of the 2,369 participants attended four or more sessions, and their average weight loss at completion was 4.7%. This approach is considered particularly effective because the CHWs are community based and able to engage people at highest risk for diabetes in a program at their local YMCA. People like attending the classes in their neighborhood, while the health care providers like it because the cost of incentivizing the CHWs to deliver the program for their enrollees is much less than treating a diabetic patient (Vojta, Koehler, Longjohn, Lever, and Caputo, 2013).

Diabetes Control

An initial review showed that half of the programs assessed for the CHW contribution to control of diabetes showed that CHWs were successful in helping patients to significantly reduce blood sugar levels (Perry, Zulliger, and Rogers, 2014). More recent studies provide additional evidence of strategies for using CHWs to help patients better manage their disease (Adair et al., 2012; Babamoto et al., 2009; Findley et al., 2014; Brown et al., 2012; Hargraves, Ferguson, Lemay, and Pernice, 2012; Heisler et al., 2009; Katula et al., 2011, 2013; Lorig, Ritter, Villa, and Armas, 2009; Otero-Sabogal et al., 2010; Prezio et al., 2013; Spencer et al., 2011; Walton, Snead, Collinsworth, and Schmidt, 2012). One of the most important studies reporting on positive CHW impact was conducted in North Carolina, where their 2-year follow-up showed that the patients enrolled in their CHWs' adaptation of the Diabetes Prevention Program had sustained reductions in weight, blood sugar, and insulin resistance, compared to those with usual care (Katula et al., 2013). For CHWs to have an impact on diabetes control, it was emphasized that both the CHW and the patient have a close relationship with the medical provider, so that they are a team in supporting the individual in the routine of checking blood sugar and taking medications as needed to control the disease (Adair et al., 2012; Heisler et al., 2009; Otero-Sabogal et al., 2010). The lack of a significant improvement in a

Massachusetts diabetes control program among patients with a CHW was attributed to poor supervision and lack of full integration of the CHW with the patient care team (Hargraves et al., 2012). The cost-effectiveness analysis of four programs including CHWs to promote self-management of diabetes showed that the programs improved the patient quality-adjusted life years (QALYs) by .30, at a cost of $39,563, well below the average expected cost of $50,000–$75,000 per QALY for resources expended to improve patient outcomes (Brownson, Hoerger, Fisher, and Kilpatrick, 2009). These results were echoed in a study focusing on the cost-effectiveness of CHWs to improve diabetes control among low-income Hispanics in Texas, which attributed to CHWs a cost-effectiveness ratio of $10,000–$33,000 per QALY gained, with the highest ratios for those with the lowest control when beginning the program (Brown et al., 2012).

Hypertension Prevention and Control

CHWs also contribute to reducing cardiovascular disease risk and hypertension (Allen et al., 2011; Balcazar, Byrd, Ortiz, Tondapu, and Chavez, 2009; Brownstein et al., 2005; Cornell et al., 2009; Fernandes et al., 2012; Harvey et al., 2009; Katula et al., 2013). As with the CHW interventions to prevent diabetes, CHWs promote a healthy diet with less fats, sugars, and salt, promoting physical activity, smoking cessation, and knowledge of hypertension symptoms and the need to check blood pressure regularly. Effectiveness has varied generally but has supported the positive contribution of CHWs, so much so that the Institute of Medicine has included a recommendation for CHWs to be a part of any community-based approach to prevent and control hypertension (Fleury, Keller, Perez, and Lee, 2009).

Asthma Self-Management

Many studies also strengthen the evidence for a positive impact of CHWs on the management of childhood asthma (Breysse et al., 2013; Bryant-Stephens, Kurian, Guo, and Zhao, 2009; Findley, Rosenthal, et al., 2011; Findley, Thomas, et al., 2011; Fisher-Owens, Boddupalli, and Thyne, 2011; Krieger, Takaro, Song, Beaudet, and Edwards, 2009; Lara et al., 2009; Margellos-Anast, Gutierrez, and Whitman, 2012; Martin, Mosnaim, Rojas, Hernandez, and Sadowski, 2011; Nelson et al., 2011; Peretz et al., 2012; Postma, Karr, and Kieckhefer, 2009). The CHWs provide education about asthma, help resolve cultural myths and tensions, coach on use of medications according to the asthma action plan, coordinate referrals for social services, encourage follow-up visits to the health care provider, and make home visits to help the family in reducing environmental triggers. The home visits that CHWs make to families with children who have asthma are an important component of the CHW success at assisting families with improving management of their children's asthma. These visits not only build the rapport between the family and the CHW, but they also ground the recommendations about asthma management and reduction of asthma triggers in the reality of their own home. This facilitates joint problem solving by the CHW and the family to take steps to reduce triggers, as well as to establish a daily asthma medication routine (Bryant-Stephens and Li, 2008; Krieger et al., 2009). Frequency of contact also contributes to the CHW's success with the family. CHWs may also complement their home visits with telephone calls to help families with problem solving, and this also may contribute to their success (Fisher-Owens et al., 2011). As with CHW support for diabetes management, it is also important for the CHW to have a strong link with the family's medical provider (Findley, Rosenthal, et al., 2011; Margellos-Anast et al., 2012; Nelson et al., 2011; Peretz et al., 2012).

Mental Health and Well-Being

Fewer studies report on the impact of CHWs to promote mental well-being, but with the adaptation of the Chronic Disease Self-Management Program (CDSMP) to train mental health peer leaders, we expect that there will be more programs in the future. The HARP program developed as an adaptation of the CDSMP showed that those with the mental health peer leader (CHW) increased patient activation and primary care visits, with some increase (not significant) in medication adherence and quality of life, compared to similar patients without the peer support (Druss et al., 2010). There is also evidence from other programs that CHWs have increased mental health service utilization (Fujiwara and Chan, 2009; Wennerstrom, 2011).

CHW programs addressing other health problems such as HIV treatment or diabetes control are beginning to incorporate activities, informal counseling, social support, and linkages to mental health services (Garcia et al., 2012; Islam et al., 2013; Ramos, Ferreria-Pinto, Rusch, and Ramos, 2010; Spencer et al., 2013). In Detroit and New York City, the CHWs helped the participants with stress reduction along with supporting them for better communication with their provider, and both showed improvements in mental well-being along with improved diabetes management behaviors (Islam et al.,

2013; Spencer et al., 2013). When CHWs were part of hospital discharge planning and followed up with patients after discharge, this resulted in patients' better mental health status post discharge and fewer readmissions within 1 month (Kangovi et al., 2014).

HIV Prevention and Treatment Adherence

There has been a long history of using peer workers to promote HIV medication adherence, both in the United States and globally, and there are some new perspectives on the use of CHWs to promote prevention or testing for HIV or adherence to HIV antiretrovirals in the United States, particularly among Latina women (Ramos et al., 2010; Sanchez, Silva-Suarez, Serna, and De La Rosa, 2012; Wingood et al., 2011). These programs emphasize the use of CHWs to facilitate development of social networks to support Latinas in confronting the realities of HIV risk.

Health Care Access and Utilization

Finally, there is increasing attention to the role of CHWs simply providing a bridge between the community and health care system, particularly for those who are the most vulnerable, with multiple chronic conditions and often the neediest in terms of health care needs. With the passage of the Affordable Care Act, there is explicit attention focused on the CHWs as the individuals most able to nurture those most vulnerable and facilitate their getting insurance and care for neglected health needs (Hawkins and Groves, 2011; Herman, 2011; Martinez Garcel, 2012; Martinez, Ro, Villa, Powell, and Knickman, 2011). Indeed, a new phrase was coined by Atul Gawande, "hot spotters," to designate how CHWs can work in the communities that are "hot spots" for multiple illnesses and heavy emergency department use (Gawande, 2011). Multiple programs are now assessing the effectiveness of CHWs to provide patient navigation or "bridging" functions to enable persons with cancer or other chronic conditions to access and use needed health and social services (Battaglia et al., 2012; Cantril and Haylock, 2013; Freeman, 2013). In addition, CHWs have been found to play a key role in enhancing continuity of care and ensuring strong patient-centered focus of primary care medical homes (Fagman et al., 2011; Findley, Matos, Hicks, Chang, and Reich, 2014; Volkmann and Castanares, 2011).

This updating of the review provides a more encouraging view of the potential for CHWs to positively contribute to promoting the health of immigrants, given the burden of chronic disease prevention faced by many immigrants, overlaid with mental health concerns and the ever-present background issues of protecting the health of their children. There is now considerable evidence of the effectiveness of CHWs for the prevention and management of diabetes, the prevention and control of hypertension, and promotion of asthma self-management. There are fewer recent studies on HIV prevention and treatment adherence, mental health and well-being, and improved health care access and utilization, but what studies do exist for these areas give promising results regarding the potential for CHWs to engage and support improved management and health care use for those in need of these services.

Evidence for Community Health Workers to Improve Immigrant Health

If CHWs are effective at improving chronic disease prevention and management among vulnerable populations, it is likely that this same approach will be beneficial for immigrant populations. This last section of the chapter reviews the evidence pertaining to this subgroup of CHW interventions, those focused on immigrants. Most of the studies concern efforts to support Latino immigrants, but there are a handful that report on the use of CHWs with other immigrant groups. Because the vast majority of studies reporting on the use of CHWs to promote immigrant health have been conducted in the United States, we exclude the half dozen that concern New Zealand, Spain, or other countries. The 77 studies included in this review were published and indexed by Medline with the key words of "community health worker," "lay health worker," "promotora," and/or "immigrant or Latino health." Most were published between 2000 and 2014, but a handful of studies are included from earlier dates. Most are comparative studies (CHW versus no CHW), some with a pre-post design, and 19 used a randomized controlled trial design. The goal for this chapter is not to definitively review the quality of evidence but to summarize how CHWs have been incorporated into programs to prevent or manage the major immigrant health problems areas and the contributions of the CHWs to resolving immigrants' health problems. Because so many of the CHW programs for immigrants are adaptations of CHW programs already discussed in the preceding section of the chapter, this discussion follows the same organization, by health problem area. In addition to summarizing the weight of the evidence concerning the relative merits of the CHW for achieving program impact, we also summarize some of the differences between the programs working with immigrants as compared to those that work with both the immigrant and US-born populations.

A summary of the programs for which CHWs were used to promote immigrant health is given in Table 2.1. The majority of the programs using CHWs to work with immigrants were focusing on chronic disease prevention or management, including both disease-specific programs and those that more broadly encouraged healthy living and prevention of multiple chronic conditions. The preponderance of programs for any single health problem area was to prevent or manage diabetes ($n = 22$, including 14 randomized controlled trial [RCT] design), followed by wellness and chronic disease prevention ($n = 7$), cancer screening and treatment ($n = 11$), cardiovascular disease prevention and control ($n = 5$, including two RCTs), HIV/STI prevention and treatment adherence ($n = 4$, including two RCTs), asthma self-management ($n = 5$, with one RCT), mental health ($n = 3$), maternal health ($n = 3$), and environmental justice ($n = 4$). If a randomized controlled trial design was not used, the studies used a pretest/posttest design to monitor changes in behavior and health outcomes with and without the CHWs, sometimes with a control group where the CHW program was not offered but to which participants were not randomly assigned.

The relative absence of studies investigating how CHWs can support maternal or child health, including child obesity prevention, breastfeeding promotion, or immunizations, may reflect the fact that these are areas that have a diverse network of maternal and child health programs funded by the federal government (e.g., prenatal care insurance, Special Supplemental Feeding program for Women, Infants, and Children [WIC], early childhood parenting programs such as Head Start), which are widely available regardless of immigrant health status. These programs may have staff who function like CHWs to support their immigrant families, but they often do not see these staff as CHWs and therefore would be less likely to examine or report on the effectiveness of their staff/CHWs. Many prenatal care programs offer nurses for care coordination, in which case CHWs might be considered superfluous, as shown in one study that added a CHW (Meghea et al., 2013). Nonetheless, focus groups with Somali immigrant women in Maine reflected many issues with prenatal care where a CHW would be invaluable for explaining delivery processes and enhancing continuity of care (Hill, Hunt, and Hyrkäs, 2012).

As will be discussed in greater detail later, all of the programs that monitored changes in participant knowledge about their health problem area and its risk factors showed that the participants with the CHWs had significant improvement in their understanding about most elements related to their

Table 2.1 CHWs and Their Roles in Promoting the Health of US Immigrants by Health Problem Area

Health Problem Area (No. of Programs)	Community Health Worker Roles and Activities	Key Elements for Immigrants	Positive Outcomes (%)
Diabetes prevention and control (22 programs, 20 with health outcomes assessed)	Outreach to individuals at risk or with poorly controlled diabetes Group and individual diabetes education, DPP or CDSMP variations Home visits and individual coaching to facilitate change Group cooking, shopping, walking activities Group and individual social support for achieving goals Promote regular blood sugar monitoring and checkups Feedback to medical provider Care coordination for social and health services Patient navigation and translation	Much attention to building trust with immigrants and their network Frequent contact between CHW and participants CHW is immigrant and bilingual, often a peer who also has diabetes Materials are bilingual and tailored for immigrant group, often with their input CHW is often given total responsibility for group and individual diabetes education Activities are community based and accepted within immigrant community Care coordination includes health insurance enrolment and legal issues CHW is conduit for communications from immigrants to help provider become more culturally sensitive	100% for knowledge, goals, or lifestyle, 85% had significant impact on A1c, BP, BMI, or LDL, though some effects not sustained
CVD prevention and control (n = 5 programs with health outcomes)	Outreach to individuals at risk for hypertension Group and individual lifestyle education (diet and activity) Group exercise/activities Group and individual support Promote regular checkups and blood pressure monitoring Promote medication adherence	CHW is immigrant and bilingual Materials bilingual and culturally tailored for immigrants, use of media Aim to enhance self-efficacy to manage chronic disease Focus on reducing fatigue and improving daily quality of life Role modeling and peers share how changed diet or activities CHW training enables them to "translate" the medical language Can be implemented in community or clinic	100% improved heart healthy diet and exercise, 100% improved cholesterol, BP or other CVD outcomes

(continued)

Table 2.1 Continued

Health Problem Area (No. of Programs)	Community Health Worker Roles and Activities	Key Elements for Immigrants	Positive Outcomes (%)
Chronic disease prevention ($n = 7$ programs, 1 with health outcomes)	Outreach to families, not just at-risk groups Group education and individual lifestyle education Group activities, especially through faith-based immigrant groups Group and individual support for positive achievements Coalition approach, with community-building events Linkage to health care system and primary care providers Patient navigation and translation	Holistic approach, addressing whole-body health Lifestyle change is the goal Culturally specific support for progressive approach to behavior change Immigrant-to-immigrant support groups Coalition approach brings in multiple stakeholders, including faith-based community Popular education approach, linking education to participant concerns Role modeling of behavior change in small increments CHW has interactive training, which builds capacity to elicit participation Supportive supervision Mutual linkage to the primary care team	100% for knowledge, screening, and behavior change indicators, 100% for health outcomes (BMI, BP, blood sugar...)
Cancer screening and care ($n = 11$ programs, 8 with outcomes)	Outreach and mobilization Motivational interviewing Group education Linkage to health care system for screening Social support and follow-up post screening Patient navigation to support timely treatment	Culturally tailored messages, delivered one-on-one by promotora Multimedia to build community awareness, but not for education Peer leaders can also promote screening and follow-up Patient navigation to support seeking care	100% increase cancer awareness and importance of testing, 100% with outcomes of CHW > no CHW
HIV/STI prevention and treatment adherence ($n = 4, 3$ with outcomes)	Outreach to women's groups or networks Home visits to at risk, with video to explain Group education and support Culturally tailored messages Facilitate testing Coaching on prevention and sexual negotiation	Outreach with immigrant women's networks Group activities link social support and education "Testing parties" hosted by immigrant women Empowerment approach to support women negotiating with men	66% increased testing

Focus area	Activities	Considerations	Outcomes
Asthma self-management (*n* = 4 programs, 3 with outcomes)	Outreach through multiple channels Group education and social support Home visits to help reduce triggers Individual coaching on appropriate use of medications Facilitate communication with provider Social support to promote adherence Link to provider for medical management	Bilingual outreach and educational materials Family approach Pictorial guides to explain medications Home visits to immigrant homes to help families reduce triggers Coaching on questions to ask provider about medications Facilitate social support from other immigrants Accompany as needed to support family in visits to provider	100% show improvement in asthma control and self-management behaviors
Mental health (*n* = 3, 2 with mental health outcomes)	Outreach to at-risk groups (elderly, single, postpartum) Group and individual social support Stress reduction activities Facilitate link to behavioral health provider	Too few studies to generalize about what works Culturally appropriate outreach Integrated into other programs Stress reduction focus Coping tips address realities of immigrant lives	100% some impact, 50% reduced depression
Maternal/infant/ nutrition (*n* = 2 programs, 2 with outcomes)	Outreach to pregnant immigrant women Group and individual education Home visits (prenatal or parenting programs) Appointment reminders Group activities with women and their children Linkage to maternal and child health services	Too few studies to generalize CHW is immigrant peer, serves as partner or mentor Bilingual materials Frequent contact from CHW to mother Dispel myths about nutrition	100% increase in recommended behaviors (reduce dietary fat or postpartum visit)
Environmental justice and advocacy (*n* = 4 programs)	Outreach for mobilization Door-to-door canvassing Participatory research Community and home visits to identify problems Stakeholder meetings Facilitate advocacy	CBPR involves individuals to also build up coalition and groups Stakeholder involvement very important CHW role models advocacy and gives social support for articulating needs and advocating for their resolution CHW is active in leading participatory research	100% increased community advocacy and involvement in environmental justice

risk for the condition, how to prevent it, and, if they already were diagnosed with the condition, how to self-manage the disease. (See Table 2.1, column 4.) The participants with the CHW support demonstrated significantly greater improvement in their health-related behaviors, such as changing some of their eating habits or making more frequent visits to their health care provider. Finally, almost all of the studies monitoring health outcomes showed significant improvement in disease prevention or control, such as reducing weight or HbA1c levels. As with the health behavior outcomes, not all health outcomes showed equal amounts of improvements. The CHW roles and activities are not dissimilar to those undertaken by CHWs in programs for both US-born and immigrant. This similarity in functions suggests that the CHWs who work in these programs do not need additional core competencies. However, as noted in column 3 of Table 2.1, the way that the CHW functions appears to be somewhat different, with more emphasis on some roles compared to others, particularly health coaching, counseling, and individualized education.

Diabetes Prevention and Control

In the last decade there has been growing public awareness of the obesity epidemic and the need to change how we live if we are to prevent diabetes and other chronic diseases, but changes in this awareness have not been universal and, as noted earlier, immigrants are likely to be those for whom the risk of chronic disease still seems far off, and certainly not as important as work or school. Thus, programs focusing on diabetes and chronic disease prevention among immigrants may not be able to start from the same base as in nonimmigrant communities. Not surprisingly, therefore, in contrast to the many recent studies of CHW effectiveness for improving diabetes prevention and control that reflected adaptations of the DPP, only two focusing on immigrants were adaptations of the DPP (Ockene et al., 2012). Most of the CHW programs for immigrants developed their own educational program as an adaptation of the American Diabetes Association recommendations for 10 weekly sessions. Some of the programs offered only individually tailored sessions, one-on-one educational sessions between the CHW and the patient, offered over a 3- to 12-month period, generally just after the patient has been diagnosed (Babamoto et al., 2009; Culica, Walton, Harker, and Prezio, 2008; Prezio et al., 2013; Rothschild et al., 2013), but the majority combined group and individual education and coaching sessions. In the combination model, the group sessions were led by certified diet educators (CDEs) or nurses (Corkery et al., 1997; Hargraves et al., 2012; Ingram,

Gallegos, and Elenes, 2005; Philis-Tsimikas, Walker, and Rivard, 2004; Thompson, Horton, and Flores, 2007), jointly led by the CDE or nurse and the CHW (Brown et al., 2012; Brown, Garcia, and Kouzekanani, 2002), or led entirely by the CHW, the case for the majority of programs (Islam et al., 2013; Joshu, Rangel, Garcia, Brownson, and O'Toole, 2007; Lorig, Ritter, and Jacquez, 2005; Lorig, Ritter, Villa, and Piette, 2008; Lujan, Ostwald, and Ortiz, 2007; Ockene et al., 2012; Palmas et al., 2012; Philis-Tsimikas, Fortmann, Lleva-Ocana, Walker, and Gallo, 2011; Spencer et al., 2011; Tang et al., 2014; Walton et al., 2012). The reliance on the CHW to lead both the group and individual sessions reflected the expectation that well-trained CHWs would provide more culturally appropriate education and seamless support in following up with the immigrants. Most of the recruitment criteria for the CHWs showed that not only were they fellow immigrants, but many also were peers, having diabetes themselves. This enhanced the ability of the CHW to model appropriate management behaviors for the participants, particularly in the individual education/coaching sessions that were included in all the CHW programs.

The effectiveness of the CHW-only model was demonstrated in all of these studies, both those with CHWs providing individual sessions only and those with CHWs leading the group and individual sessions. Indeed, two of the three studies with negative results for the CHW intervention were those where the CHW only followed up with immigrants after education by a CDE or nurse (Corkery et al., 1997; Hargraves et al., 2012). The CHW-only programs attained significant reductions in HbA1c (marker for blood sugar levels) after participating in the program, and if analyzed in detail, the greatest reductions occurring for those with higher HbA1c levels at enrollment (Hargraves et al., 2012), women and older participants (Babamoto et al., 2009; Thompson et al., 2007), those with higher levels of participation in the program (>80% completion rate; Corkery et al., 1997; Culica et al., 2008; Ingram et al., 2005), or with greater numbers of CHW contacts or duration of assistance (Islam et al., 2013; Lujan et al., 2007; Ockene et al., 2012; Philis-Tsimikas et al., 2011; Rothschild et al., 2013). Other positive outcomes for the CHW model observed in various studies were improved self-reported health status, increased exercise levels and fruit and vegetable consumption, weight loss, reduced blood pressure, greater medication adherence, reduced depression or distress; and reduced urgent care visits (Babamoto et al., 2009; Culica et al., 2008; Hargraves et al., 2012; Ingram et al., 2005; Lorig et al., 2005; Ockene et al., 2012; Rothschild et al., 2013; Ruggiero et al., 2011; Spencer et al., 2013; Tang et al., 2014; Thompson et al., 2007).

Compared to the CHW programs not specifically targeting immigrant groups, the immigrant-focused programs emphasized the training of CHWs in core competencies of trust building, communication, counseling, and providing social support. In virtually all the programs, the CHWs were immigrants or had the same cultural background, and many were selected because they were peers, people with diabetes under control. (See Table 2.1, column 3.) By giving the CHW a role in education and coaching about diabetes, they promoted more trust between the CHW and the participants. This was reinforced by frequent contacts, with combined education and follow-up contacts averaging more than the monthly level seen in many CHW interventions. Another distinguishing feature of these programs is the use of a participatory approach to developing the materials and CHW support program, so that the program and its materials were tailored by and for the specific immigrant groups with whom the CHW would be working. Some adapted the Chronic Care Model so that it appropriately reflected support for issues unique to the immigrant population regarding access to and confidence in the health care system. Although some CHWs were based at collaborating clinics, the majority of the group education sessions were held at community organizations, churches, schools, and other settings readily accessible to the immigrants. In ensuring that the patients maintained contact with the health care team, the CHWs also facilitated enrollment into insurance programs or explained how their care would be covered at the facility. Finally, the CHW provided feedback to and from the health care team, so that when the immigrants went for their diabetes care they would have a more satisfying encounter with the provider.

Cardiovascular Disease Prevention and Control

The programs integrating CHWs for cardiovascular health among immigrants ($n = 5$ programs) also have been effective, though not across all heart disease markers. The most well-known program, Salud Para Su Corazon, a collaboration between the researchers, community organizations on the Texas-Mexican border, the National Heart, Lung, and Blood Institute, and the Health Resources Services Administration. CHWs changed attitudes and perceptions regarding cardiovascular risk factors, and they were associated with advancing dietary changes such as reduced fat and salt intake, increasing exercise, facilitating weight loss, and reducing LDL cholesterol and blood pressure (Balcázar, 2009; Balcázar et al., 2009). The Salud Para Su Corazon program of eight educational sessions is delivered by trained

CHWs using culturally appropriate materials and approaches. The CHWs were equally effective if the sessions were offered at community organizations or at collaborating clinics (Balcázar, 2011). The Salud Para Su Corazon has been adopted as a national recommendation from the CDC. The NHLBI/HRSA collaboration included a team in Hawaii that developed a Healthy Heart, Healthy Family program offered by Filipino CHWs to Filipino families in Hawaii. This program also showed a significant improvement in knowledge about heart disease, importance of diet and exercise, and improvement in self-efficacy to change behavior. The CHW intervention led to lower cholesterol (total and LDL) and lower blood sugar, but there were no reductions in blood pressure, BMI, or waist circumference, which actually increased (Fernandes et al., 2012). The other two CHW interventions focused on promoting blood pressure and diabetes screening, along with a provision of information about healthy eating, and both were effective at reaching Latinos through the Healthy Connections "house parties" (Harvey et al., 2009) and South Asian immigrants through "camps" (Gany, Levy, Basu, and Misra, 2012).

As with the diabetes prevention and control programs discussed earlier, the cardiovascular disease prevention and management programs employing CHWs to work with immigrant populations focused on community-based activities, held at churches or other social settings where immigrants would be comfortable. (See Table 2.1, column 3.) Materials were all bilingual and culturally tailored for immigrants, backed up by radio spots in some cases. They introduced novel ways to reach and engage immigrants, for example, house parties or "camps," much like community health fairs. The programs focused much more on building self-efficacy to manage disease and make improvements to the individual's daily life. Instead of focusing on disease control, the focus in these programs tended to be positive, on health and improving daily quality of life. The peer CHWs were effective at showing that making changes, such as to diet, were feasible, because they had done it themselves. Importantly, the CHW helped people understand the medical language and reduced fears about the disease.

Chronic Disease Prevention

Several of the CHW programs for immigrants ($n = 7$) were developed to promote healthy lifestyles more generally, not just to prevent diabetes or hypertension alone, but only two report on behavioral or health outcomes, both positively (Grigg-Saito et al., 2010; Hunter et al., 2004). Four programs describe how input from community organizations and immigrants them-selves helped them to create a program truly responsive to the needs and situa-tion of immigrants (Drieling, Ma, and Stafford, 2011; Grigg-Saito et al., 2010; Han, Kim, and Kim, 2007; Messias et al., 2013). Through the involvement of multiple organizations, health provider groups, and religious leaders, a pro-gram to promote "Whole Community" among Cambodian immigrants in Massachusetts was able to reach many segments of the Cambodian popula-tion. Outcomes were also monitored across partners and included changes in diet habits, more HIV awareness, reduced depression, improved communica-tion with health providers, and increased blood pressure and blood glucose control (Grigg-Saito et al., 2010). Another study documented the importance of tailoring chronic health promotion interventions to the specific needs of the immigrant community, in this case Koreans and Korean Americans (Han et al., 2007). Another recommended change to program structure was to close the disconnects between the diabetes educators and the promotoras, where the diabetes educators not fully appreciated the work of the promoto-ras while the promotoras were unaware of the procedures or resources avail-able at the clinic (Keller, Borges, Hoke, and Radasa, 2011).

Compared to other programs utilizing CHWs for chronic disease pre-vention, the programs focusing on immigrants were more likely to take a more holistic approach, including diagnosis and assistance with depression and stress. Their message was more positive and general, aiming for a healthy lifestyle. Programs were carefully adapted to the needs and situation of the immigrants, as in the program for Cambodian immigrants in Massachusetts. Several incorporated immigrant-to-immigrant support groups, reaching across partner organizations. The CHWs worked closely with faith-based organizations, and this appears to have enhanced their trust and hence their reach into the community. When working with immigrants, the CHW used popular education approaches, interactively linking education to participant concerns. They were trained in and demonstrated the possibility of behavioral change in small, feasible increments. As with the other CHW programs work-ing with immigrants, these programs also recommended strong links between the CHW and the primary care team, with frequent supportive supervision.

Cancer Screening and Treatment

Cancer screening among immigrants is particularly challenging, because in addition to fears about cancer carried over from their home countries, the immigrants may have additional fears about interacting with the health care system, including both fear of deportation and fear about cost due to lack of insurance. Therefore, the promotoras who support cancer screening and treatment promotion as patient navigators do much more than simply reminding and navigating. They also help women understand about breast and/or cervical cancer, dispel their fears about screening, help resolve cultural barriers to self-examination and prevention, and help them understand that screening is a positive contribution to their lives and their ability to serve their families. They also help them understand the results, help them to get any further tests needed to diagnose their condition, and then help them with appointments so they receive prompt treatment. All eight of the breast and/or cervical cancer screening programs for underserved Latina or immigrant women had significant increases in breast and/or cancer screening rates, approximately double the rates without patient navigation (Calderon et al., 2010; Fernandez et al., 2009; Mock et al., 2007; Navarro, Raman, McNicholas, and Loza, 2007; Nuno, Martinez, Harris, and Garcia, 2011; Percac-Lima, Ashburner, Bond, Oo, and Atlas, 2013; Raich, Whitley, Thorland, Valverde, and Fairclough, 2012; Wells et al., 2012).

Critical to the patient navigator/promotora's success is tailoring messages carefully to address different views about cancer risk and survivability, often using a social learning or stages of change model (Fernandez et al., 2009; Ramirez et al., 2014; Wells et al., 2012). The application of the stages of change model was effective at reducing the time to treatment among Latinas with breast cancer (Ramirez et al., 2014). Media raised awareness of cancer risk in the immigrant community (Wells et al., 2012), but educational videos appear to have little additional impact beyond the personal interactions with the CHW (Calderon et al., 2010; Mock et al., 2007). Cancer survivors can also be used to promote screening, but they need different training than CHWs who are not also cancer survivors, as these different groups have different underlying understandings about cancer (Saad-Harfouche et al., 2011).

HIV/STI Prevention and Treatment Adherence

Only four studies were identified that used CHWs to promote HIV/STI prevention, testing, and/or treatment adherence (Ramos et al., 2010; Sanchez et al., 2012; Taylor et al., 2009; Wingood et al., 2011). The Spread the Word program among immigrants in Texas and New Mexico used a social network approach and introduced "testing parties" held in different women's homes, with which the CHW support increased counseling and rapid testing to 50%

of the participants (Ramos et al., 2010). The AMIGAS program also used CHW-led group sessions to successfully promote consistent condom use and its negotiation among Latinas. They used an empowerment approach to give women stronger negotiating skills with men (Wingood et al., 2011). An individual approach was used for CHWs working with Chinese Americans and Chinese immigrants to the United States and Canada, who watched a video together with the CHW and then went to the clinic for Hepatitis B testing. These visits increased Hepatitis B knowledge and self-reported testing, but not all tests were confirmed by medical providers (Taylor et al., 2009).

Asthma Self-Management

The asthma self-management programs all focus on families with young children (typically aged 2–10 years) who have asthma. The CHW programs for immigrant families build on earlier child asthma management programs, such as Yes We Can, the National Inner City Asthma Study, and Allies Against Asthma (Friedman et al., 2006; Mitchell et al., 2005; Thyne, Rising, Legion, and Love, 2006). With immigrant families the emphasis has been on explaining that asthma is manageable to parents who are panicked about their child's coughing and wheezing, and then to explain what they have to do to follow the doctor's recommendations to get the child's asthma under control (Martin et al., 2011). This entails cultural translation to inform about asthma and then suggestions on how to include managing a child's chronic illness as part of parenting (Nelson et al., 2012). CHWs have used pictorial guides or bilingual videos to help them in educating and coaching parents about their child's medications. Given the complicated nature of managing a child's asthma medications, the CHW programs for asthma self-management all have strong links to health care providers, and most include a care coordination element that is managed by the CHW. These care coordination programs have adopted a family approach, recognizing that the parents' ability to manage a young child's asthma may require resolving some of the larger problems the family faces, such as housing or job security or the need to find child care (Fox et al., 2007; Lara et al., 2013; Lob, Boer, Porter, Núñez, and Fox, 2011; Peretz et al., 2012). In addition, CHWs also work with families through home visits to reduce the children's exposure to indoor allergens and other environmental asthma triggers, often including such items as dust covers for mattresses, integrated pest management programs, and smoking cessation for adult members of the family (Postma et al., 2009). Thus, the

CHWs are called to perform a wide variety of tasks, in close partnership with the medical care team. The evidence shows that they have been successful in this multitasking. All the programs with outcomes reported significant reductions in the child's asthma symptoms, in urgent care or emergency department visits, and in hospitalizations (Fox et al., 2007; Lara et al., 2013; Lob et al., 2011; Peretz et al., 2012).

Mental Health

Only three studies reported on CHWs promoting mental health among immigrants, and only two of them reported outcomes in terms of reduced stress, depression, or mental health. Both used a patient empowerment or popular education approach to increase social capital and reduce immigrants' stress and sense of isolation (Michael, Farquhar, Wiggins, and Green, 2008; Spencer et al., 2013). The CHWs were effective in building social support, particularly through places of worship (Michael et al., 2008); the empowerment model was associated with reduced disease-related stress, but no reduction in depression (Spencer, Hawkins, Espitia, et al., 2013). The Project Wings program in Minnesota aims to reduce stress and depression among Latino adolescents and their families through CHW home visits, but no results are as yet reported (Garcia et al., 2012). While there are too few studies upon which to assess lessons learned in how CHWs help immigrants reduce stress and improve their mental well-being, the few studies all use an empowerment approach, aimed at combatting isolation, building social capital and helping the families support each other in taking steps to reduce stress and loneliness. The other important feature of these programs is that they are embedded into other programs, such as school or church, so that mental health concerns are not singled out where they can be potentially stigmatizing or, conversely, ignored as "unimportant" or socially taboo.

Maternal Health and Nutrition

Although there is great interest in incorporating CHWs for the promotion of maternal, newborn, and child health in Africa and Asia, in the United States there are only two studies reporting on CHW programs focusing on maternal health among immigrants, and these focus on the mother's health. The Secretos de la Buena Vida program in San Diego, California, employed CHWs to lead group education sessions for which the participants had weekly homework assignments, the latter also serving as an incentive, since completed assignments qualified the participant for the weekly program raffle. While the CHW classes did facilitate dietary changes to reduce fat intake, the addition of the weekly newsletter enhanced the CHW effect (Baquero et al., 2009). The other program, Prenatal Partners in Phoenix, Arizona, resembled more closely the traditional prenatal care program, with the CHW meeting with women during their pregnancy to promote a healthy infant. In addition, they found that the more visits with the Prenatal Partner, the more likely a woman was to have a postpartum visit and subsequent wellness visits (Marsiglia, Bermudez-Parsai, and Coonrod, 2010).

Environmental Justice

The history of the CHW movement is one that includes a strong role for the CHW as an advocate for the community, both for patient rights within the health system but also for the community to advocate for its collective rights, such as protections from predatory landlords or toxic chemicals from industries in or near the neighborhood, or other environmental injustices (Balcazar et al., 2011; Lara, Akinbami, Flores, and Morgenstern, 2006). This tradition is continued with four programs where CHWs work with coalitions of the immigrant communities to strengthen the *community's* capacity to prioritize and advocate for its needs through policy and legislative action: Poder es Salud/Power for Health in Portland, Oregon (Farquhar and Michael, 2004; Farquhar et al., 2008; Wiggins et al., 2009); La Red de Asma Infantil in Puerto Rico (Lara et al., 2013); Si Se Puede in San Diego, California (Minkler, Garcia, Williams, LoPresti, and Lilly, 2010), and the San Diego Mid-City collaborative (O'Neill, Williams, and Reznik, 2008). The distinguishing features of these programs are that they are all community-based participatory research studies, a partnership of academic and community organizations in which the CHWs play leading roles in networking with immigrant communities, engaging them in dialogue, and then supporting them in prioritizing issues and developing advocacy approaches to neighborhood, city, and state officials. Unlike many of the CHW programs that focus on changing health one by one, immigrant by immigrant, the environmental justice programs work with the entire community to advocate for system-wide changes that will benefit all in the community. While this has included health system changes, these programs have included a variety of environmental justice initiatives. The Si Se Puede program built advocacy for regulations to improve, among other things, the entire ambient air of the community, through advocating for regulations controlling siting and emission of toxic waste (Minkler et al., 2010). The San Diego Mid-City collaborative strove for a more functional partnership across multiple agencies to promote community development, reduce violence, and improve safety (O'Neill et al., 2008). Both the Si Se Puede and La Red de Asma Infantil addressed housing and air quality issues as part of their approach to systemwide changes to reduce the burden of asthma in their communities. In all these programs, the CHWs were more involved with advocacy and participatory research than in many of the other programs discussed earlier.

Conclusions: The Potential for Community Health Workers to Promote Immigrant Health

The studies reviewed in this chapter show that CHWs can play a strong role in promoting the health of immigrants. There is abundant evidence from around the world and across many cultures that CHWs are effective at improving health outcomes, particularly in prevention of illness, both infectious and chronic disease. CHWs work with groups or one on one with individuals, teaching them how they can take steps to protect themselves and their children from disease, whether by going to the clinic to have their children immunized or by changing their diet and activity patterns to lower the risk of diabetes. CHWs also teach people how to use the medications and treatments prescribed by their health care provider. Whether to treat a sick child with diarrhea or with asthma, the CHWs have helped parents know what medicine to use and how to give it so that their child regains health. While with additional training CHWs have been able to help people take lifesaving medications in the case of emergencies, the more important role played by CHWs is to sensitize people to the danger signs in themselves or their family that mean that they must go to the clinic right away. CHWs also help people manage medications and lifestyle changes needed to self-manage and control their chronic diseases, whether asthma, diabetes, hypertension, HIV/AIDS, or mental health. What distinguishes the CHW from the nurse or social worker are the shared life experiences, peer relationship and hands-on approach through which the CHW connects with and supports the individual to make the changes in his or her daily or weekly routine that will allow the individual to become adherent to the regimen recommended by his or her health care provider. Because the CHW shares a set of life experiences (perhaps including language and cultural heritage), even if not from the same community, the CHW can explain things in ways that the people understand. From this insider perspective, the CHW can also help people problem-solve to find ways to adapt their lifestyle or daily routines to be able to do what they have to do to stay healthy.

These same processes serve them well in working with immigrants. As our review of primarily US-based studies shows, CHWs have worked with immigrants in nine basic health problem areas: diabetes prevention and control, cardiovascular disease prevention and control, general chronic disease prevention, cancer screening and care, HIV/STI prevention and treatment adherence, asthma self-management, mental health, maternal and child health, and environmental justice/advocacy. For each of these program areas, but particularly for the first three related to prevention and control of diabetes, hypertension, and other chronic diseases, CHWs have been effective at helping people to better understand chronic diseases and what they can do to prevent or self-manage them through lifestyle changes, resulting in improved control of these chronic diseases. CHWs working with immigrants also have been effective at improving asthma prevention and control, as well as at promoting cancer screening and HIV/AIDS prevention and treatment adherence. Although CHWs traditionally have had a strong role in promoting environmental justice for their communities, this was the focus of reports from only four programs, perhaps reflecting the difficulty of funding environmental justice studies. All four studies reported increased community participation in advocacy for environmental justice. There were very few studies that examined how CHWs promote mental or maternal and child health among immigrants, but these are also areas where CHWs have supported immigrant families.

The program descriptions highlight several features that enable the CHWs to work effectively with immigrants. First, the CHWs are often immigrants themselves, and if not immigrants, they are often second-generation immigrants and have a set of shared life experiences, perhaps including language, culture, and community. This enables them to build trust with the immigrants, and develop relationships based on experience and hope rather than just theory or knowledge, which is enhanced by materials that are tailored by and for the immigrant community. Thus, immigrants can relate easily to the CHWs and any materials the CHWs use to support communications. Second, CHWs are given responsibility for leading educational, support or discussion groups with the immigrants. Successful programs have developed an educational approach that is respectful of the participants, engaging them as adult learners and facilitating interactive participatory learning. This appears to facilitate greater trust and participation among the immigrants, who appear to do less well when nurses or other trained health workers lead these groups. With the CHW leading, they appear to be more likely to speak up and support each other. These exchanges within the group build social support for behavioral changes being promoted by the CHWs, further reinforcing the message that change is possible. Third, the CHWs support the immigrants holistically, not just on the specific health problem area for which they have primary responsibility. This holistic approach is reinforced by popular education techniques used by several programs, whereby the participants set their own goals and agendas for change, which can include a wide range of issues, not just health related. Depending on these goals, CHWs help immigrants with legal issues, including housing or immigrant status issues, obtaining insurance for which they are qualified, or referrals for social services. That the CHWs often work within the context of a school, community center, or faith-based community enhances this understanding that the CHW is there for the community, not just for one health issue. Fourth, the CHWs appear to be more effective when they are nested within a system of supportive supervision, with adequate training and support to give them confidence to not only work in the community but to be viewed by the health care team as "their" community representative, a feature identified as critical to success by several programs addressing diabetes, chronic disease prevention, and asthma management. Fifth, the CHWs do appear to function as a bridge between the immigrant community and the medical providers and the larger health system. While some of the programs are structured as patient navigator programs where CHWs may focus primarily on making appointments and helping patients manage care across multiple providers and clinics, in most cases the translational aspects of the CHWs' work go far beyond simple patient navigation or translation. Their materials and educational sessions with immigrants are critical to helping the immigrants understand what the doctor really wants them to do. In some programs, the CHWs are also conduits of information back to the medical providers, helping them to improve their interactions with immigrants, if not linguistically at least culturally, to be respectful and understanding of the immigrant's cultural beliefs and fears related to his or her health problem.

Returning to Anna's dream, we conclude that this is a dream worth pursuing. CHWs are well suited to bridge the gap between immigrants and the health care system. We already have begun to build experience in integrating CHWs for the promotion of immigrant health, and the existing studies suggest that this can reach more immigrants and give them the opportunities to improve their health outcomes, particularly in the arena of chronic disease prevention and management, which is the greatest challenge faced by immigrants.

3

Becoming a Community
Health Worker

WHEN WE THINK about influential people in our lives, we tend to think of our immediate family, namely our parents, aunts, or grandparents, or of teachers or leaders who made a mark on us, such as a favorite teacher from high school, the Girl Scouts leader, a spiritual leader, or a team captain. These people inspired us, showed us a different way to think that continues to echo within us as we make our way in the world. Talking with community health workers (CHWs), it is clear that they aspire to being influential, to inspiring change among the people they serve. Depending on your perspective, the CHW's role might be in between sister and coach. They want to be that role model, teacher, or source of insight that helps the proverbial light bulb come on in people's heads as they reflect on their options. To have this influence on people, it takes a special kind of person, complemented by training in using their personal strength to connect with people and help them to make changes. This chapter focuses on how CHWs become these influential people.

We start the chapter by defining who CHWs are and then provide a global perspective on the number of people who now consider themselves to be CHWs. Then, we address the question, "Who makes the best CHWs?" describing the character attributes that underpin the ability to be a CHW. Even with the right attributes, however, it takes training and experience to shape these attributes into the person who is a CHW. Informed by the surveys we have conducted among CHWs in New York, the next section of the chapter discusses how people become CHWs, that is, the roles or activities that they are trained to master in order to actually influence and facilitate change in others' lives. Where the CHWs working with immigrants need additional skills or capabilities, we will highlight those differences in the discussion. The different attributes and skills, as well as the transformative processes experienced as people become CHWs, will be illustrated with personal accounts from the dozens of CHWs we interviewed for this book.

Who Are Community Health Workers? Global and Local Perspectives

A profession that is at once ancient and emerging, the CHW model has its roots in the natural evolution of individuals dedicated to helping others overcome health disparities and related economic and social inequities. CHWs have existed in human communities throughout history. In both the United States and the developing world, the CHW model has became formalized in areas where large sectors of the population lack health care and the conditions for good health (Wiggins, 2012). Attention was drawn to CHWs by the Chinese barefoot doctors of the 1950s, at about the same time when CHWs also were becoming involved in community development programs in the United States (Lehmann and Sanders, 2007; Rosenthal, 1998). From the 1950s through the 1970s, in both the United States and in selected Asian, Latin American, and African nations, CHWs played a strong health advocacy role, linking health promotion to community development and poverty eradication programs (Lehmann and Sanders, 2007; Werner and Bower 2012). After the Alma Ata 1978 declaration proposing national CHW programs as part of the goal of achieving health for all, since the 1980s globally CHWs have become more focused on health promotion, with more training and formal linkages to the primary health care system. With the worldwide economic recession, CHWs became part of governmental strategies to provide health care for all at lower cost. Indeed, CHWs have been described as the only "feasible and acceptable link between the health sector and the community that can be developed to meet the goal of improved health in the near term" (Kahssay, Taylor, and Berman 1998, p. 5), and they often serve as the first point of contact for families living far from any health facility (Singh and CHW Technical Task Force, 2011).

With this evolution into roles with more explicit health content, their titles have become more diversified, often including in their title the condition on which the particular CHW most focuses (see Fig. 3.1).

Community health worker,
Community health worker, community follow-up workers, community health advocates,
Community health advisers, community health aides,
Community health extension workers, community health outreach workers, community health promoter, community health representatives, community health specialists, community health volunteer,
Counselors,
Family support workers, family health promoters,
Health extension worker, Health advisors, health facilitators, health information specialists,
Health promoters, health liaisons, health specialists, case worker,
HIV counselors, HIV/STD prevention counselors, HIV risk assessment/disclosure counselors,
Lay health worker, mental health aides, nutrition assistants, bare foot doctor,
Navigators, patient navigators,
Outreach workers, outreach specialists, prenatal health specialists,
Peer counselors, peer educators, peer health advisors, peer health educators,
peer workers,
Promotoras,
Public health advisors, public service aides,
Social worker assistants, rural health motivator,
Village health worker, volunteers, women's health specialists.

FIGURE 3.1 What CHW are called.

Beginning in the early 2000s and with the push for achievement of the Healthy People 2010 goals, paralleling the setting of the Millennium Development Goals for 2015, CHWs have been identified as critical front-line public health workers. In 2009, the Community Health Worker Section (CHW Section) obtained approval from the American Public Health Association for the following definition for a community health worker, submitted for use by the Bureau of Labor Statistics for the 2010 Standard Occupation Classification revision prior to the 2010 Census:

> Community Health Workers (CHWs) are frontline public health workers who are trusted members of and/or have an unusually close understanding of the community served. This trusting relationship enables CHWs to serve as a liaison/link/intermediary between health/social services and the community to facilitate access to services and improve the quality and cultural competence of service delivery. CHWs also build individual and community capacity by increasing health knowledge and self-sufficiency through a range of activities such as outreach, community education, informal counseling, social support, and advocacy. (APHA 2009)

The Bureau of Labor Statistics approved the following definition for the tasks of CHWs (SOC# 21-1094):

Assist individuals and communities to adopt healthy behaviors. Conduct outreach for medical personnel or health organizations to implement programs in the community that promote, maintain, and improve individual and community health. May provide information on available resources, provide social support and informal counseling, advocate for individuals and community health needs, and provide services such as first aid and blood pressure screening. May collect data to help identify community health needs. (US Department of Labor, 2009, p. 3923)

Parallel efforts were led by the Global Health Workforce Alliance for a definition of CHWs that could be used to anchor efforts by countries to scale up CHWs as part of their national health workforce. Key to the global efforts was to synchronize under the CHW banner both volunteer and remunerated health providers who work within and among the community. Based on their view of the CHW as an extension of the primary health care system, the GHWA defines CHWs as follows:

CHWs should be members of the communities where they work, should be selected by the communities, should be answerable to the communities for their activities, should be supported by the health system but not necessarily a part of its organization, and have shorter training than professional workers. (Bhutta et al., 2010, p. 17)

How Many Community Health Workers?

The World Health Organization (WHO) estimates that there are approximately 1.3 million CHWs, both paid and unpaid. This includes many CHWs who work with community organizations who do report CHWs, but it is very possible that the number worldwide could be higher than the estimated 1.3 million, as many programs may not report CHW employment to the health system (World Health Organization [WHO], 2013). There is very incomplete reporting of CHWs, and some countries do not have any systematic accounting for CHWs, even though it is known that such programs exist in their countries. Others place the number of CHWs globally to be closer to 5 million (Perry, Zulliger, and Rogers, 2014).

Estimates of the number of CHWs in the United States also range widely, from 80,000 to 200,000 (Perry et al., 2014). The 2007 National Workforce Study of CHWs estimated that there were approximately 120,000 CHWs in the United States in 2005, with an estimated 11,000 CHWs in New York (US Department of Health and Human Services, 2007). This was considered an "upper bound" estimate, produced using an approach as inclusive as possible of occupations that might be interpreted as involving community health work. Applying the newly adopted BLS definition for CHW, the Bureau of Labor Statistics reports a total of 45,800 CHWs employed in the United States as of May 2013, with California, Texas, Illinois, New York, and Florida being the states with the most employed CHWs. In contrast to the locations of CHWs globally in rural communities, the majority of the US CHWs are working in metropolitan areas: Chicago, Los Angeles, New York, Philadelphia, Baltimore, Boston, Washington, DC, San Diego, San Francisco, and Sacramento (US Department of Labor, 2014).

Why Become a Community Health Worker?

Globally, the people who become CHWs are more likely to be female than male. In their 2007 survey of CHWs, Lehmann and Sanders (2007) found across multiple countries that 70% were female and 18% both male and female. This reflects the types of programs for which they are recruited to work in low-income rural settings: to promote reproductive, newborn, maternal, and child health, all of which involves work with mothers (Lassi, Majeed, Rashid, Yakoob, and Bhutta, 2013; Tran et al., 2014). Because women are often uncomfortable and sometimes prohibited from allowing men to visit them in their homes, there is a distinctive preference for women, particularly in Muslim-dominated societies such as Bangladesh, Pakistan, Ethiopia, Somalia, and Nigeria. There is also a preference for "mature" women, who are married and at least in their mid-twenties. Although the Anglophone countries have training programs for community health extension workers (CHEWs), until recently in most countries these trained CHEWs work only in clinical settings as facility-based primary health care workers, with little actual outreach and community-based health promotion. With the exception of the CHEWs who have been recruited and hired to work as salaried CHWs providing community-based service delivery, globally the majority of CHWs are recruited by the community, most as volunteers or with small stipends. They generally receive a practical, skills-oriented training of a few days to a month, just prior to beginning their service (Lehmann and Sanders, 2007; Tran et al., 2014).

The demographic profile of CHWs in New York is not dissimilar to that found globally. Our survey of the CHWs in New York ($n = 223$) shows that the majority (78%) of the CHWs are women, with an average age of 38.7 years. Most are Latino (59%), then African/African American (26%), and the balance Asian and Caucasian. Just under half (42%) are immigrants themselves. Compared to US-born CHWs, the immigrant CHWs are less likely to be female (73% versus 80%), to be Latino (55% versus 63%), and more likely to be African or African American (36.6% versus 17.4%). Half had a high school diploma or less education, and only 10% had a college degree. Regardless of immigrant status, 88% are currently working as a CHW, and they had been working at their current job for an average of 4.3 years. More of the immigrant CHWs are working for hourly wages (55% versus 41%) than the US-born CHWs and fewer had salaried positions (40% versus 51%). Unlike their counterparts in other countries, only 6% of US-born CHWs are volunteers.

The primary reasons why people became CHWs are to work with people (76%) and to work for their community (71%). Half said they became a CHW to give back to the community (54%) or to address health concerns important to the CHW or his or her family (52%). Very few CHWs said that they were working as a CHW simply because it was a job they could get (6%). As shown in Figure 3.2, immigrant CHWs are motivated by the same primary concerns

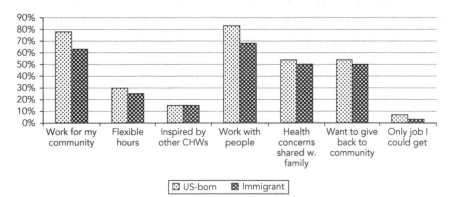

FIGURE 3.2 Why became a community health worker by immigrant status, New York CHW Survey 2008–2010.

as other CHWs, but they appear to be less clear about their motivation than US-born CHWs. For practically every reason, fewer immigrant CHWs gave any response compared to the US-born. This suggests that there may be other factors affecting their choice.

We heard again and again of the CHWs' deep-seated urge to work with people, to help those who are suffering. Gordon, a second-generation Jamaican working with the city's visiting nurse service as a case manager, spoke about why he became a CHW. He also spoke about the importance of a shared cultural and ethnic background, which helps him in his work.

I've always had an affinity for helping people, but it really started when I was trying to understand why minority homosexual men use crystal meth. It was really interesting to hear the reasoning, like some of them wanted to fit in, some of them felt freer when they used it, it was just interesting to see the mechanisms for the use and also to see how it played its role in causing them to have such a high rate of HIV, so I think that's when it started. I wanted to make a difference and that led me to become a CHW. It came naturally for me. Being a minority, in terms of being Black, helps me to meet my clients at where they are at. In terms of speaking/communicating with them, it's not a by-the-book, textbook interaction. I can adjust myself, the way I speak to who I'm speaking to, because I've experienced being a minority and know where they are coming from.

Working for one's own community is the other dominant reason why most people become CHWs, regardless of their own immigrant status. Like the majority of CHWs motivated by wanting to work in the community, a young man from Chicago demonstrated how wanting to work with his own community to help people led him toward becoming a CHW.

My interest was initially to work with immigrants, and I was not interested specifically in health issues. In the area where I live about 30% of the population is Hispanic, mainly undocumented. I wanted to get involved in that community in some way. I had an interest in finding out more about the psychological issues immigrants face in my community. Even though I did not have any training in health, a very good opportunity came up. So, becoming a mental health facilitator has helped me to approach and help a lot of people in the community.

The desire to give back to the community of immigrants was echoed by several CHWs, particularly in combination with a desire to help others avoid the pain they had experienced as immigrants, as these five immigrant CHWs remarked.

I've been in New York for 10 years, but I also worked in Florida, also with the immigrant population. What inspired me to become a community health worker is the need that I saw in the immigrant community, of people not knowing how to navigate the system, not knowing what are their rights, and the barrier of the language as well as the health literacy.

When I was pregnant, I felt isolated, without any community support. In my own country, Jordan, the community is very involved with a woman's pregnancy and postpartum care. So, I wanted to do this here, I wanted to help other pregnant women so they would not be alone.

They [Alianza] helped me with everything. They gave me favor and treated me well, so now I want to give back. There are so many people with great need, and all around here people are caring, it is all about helping each other. So, if I have an opportunity to help someone, I must do it. I am so grateful for everything.

I have had my own personal struggles, to have money for food and clothing. I felt I wanted to give back to the community, and I was drawn to this work because I felt that I was already a good caregiver.

I knew that Alianza was basically an organization to help immigrants, and when I finished the AA degree I thought of Alianza as an organization where I could serve the community and start my career in human services. So I called them and they had an opening for a male CHW. I was attracted by the opportunity to assist those in need, as well as applying certain knowledge and people skills acquired at work and in the academic sphere.

Being a good CHW means being a good networker. Those who naturally try to make connections with and between others naturally are drawn to the work. We hear again from Karime, who is a CHW and advocate for the West African community in New York City.

It is a matter of vision and mission. I see it as an opportunity to empower the community. That is very appealing to me. I became a CHW because I like being able to connect community members to the services they need.

As a CHW, it gives me more possibility to link to people. I can use my own experience to help them. Culturally, I am familiar with growing up in the West African culture and being a Muslim that is also important as many of the immigrants I work with are Muslim. This combination of factors makes it easy for me to connect with everyone.

Many spoke of the importance of creating linkages or ties between fellow immigrants and the health system, to help them know their rights and help them get what they are entitled to, as these two immigrants said.

I wanted to build linkages between the community and medical care. I wanted work that would make a difference, help people "take off" and achieve goals. I liked the idea of being a CHW also because of the interaction, making friends with clients.

I've done this work all of my life. I always defended my classmates if they were wrongly accused. I had a lovely seventh-grade teacher in the Bronx, and she saw me do this. She gave me a law book and told me someday I'd be somebody. I've made it my business to know where we can receive benefits for my community. I've been doing this my entire life. It feels so good to help people. Even if it doesn't work out for the person, it feels good to have tried to help.

For some of the immigrants, becoming a CHW was the natural thing to do after seeing their parents being CHWs themselves back in their home country. We hear again from Lucinda, whose mother was a CHW in El Salvador.

I think that a lot in my past life prepared me for my work. I grew up in El Salvador during the civil war, and I was always concerned about justice and equality, helping people. My mother is a natural community health worker, because she is always the person who helped the people in the *colonia* where we lived. If there was a drunk person on the street, she would give them a plate of food. So, I had a huge influence from my mother, who was always helping people. People have big needs and little resources, but from her I learned that it is possible to do something. After high school [in Rochester] I went to a community college and was thinking of different things I wanted to do and I like helping people. I did some volunteer work, and I really liked it. I wanted to get a degree in social work, but I could not go to school and work full time and still do the fieldwork hours. Then, I realized that as a community health worker I still could help others. It was during my first summer job, tutoring children. I also worked with their parents, and I did home visits as part of that job, to see how the family could be more supportive to their children's studies. Making these visits, I was hooked. This was what I wanted to do. It got me out of the office, and I could follow through with people. I really liked it. I am glad now that I did not become a social worker. I have more freedom to be creative with what I do as a community health worker than if I had gone into social work.

Our survey showed that half the CHWs said they became a CHW because they wanted to do something about a health problem their family was experiencing. We hear again from Arelia about her experience with a sick nephew, having to learn how to care for his asthma, and then realizing that she wanted to be a CHW.

It started off because my nephew got asthma when he was 2. My nephew lived with me since he was born, and it was hard for me to grasp what was happening. Doctors gave us a bunch of medications, and I was doing everything that the doctor said. But he was very sick, and I gave him too many pumps because I just wanted him to stop coughing, and then he overdosed and had to go to the ER. So, I learned all about asthma, and gradually I learned how to control it better. I needed to learn about the disease, go to the library to use the computer, so I could ask the doctor questions. I kept thinking: Why did I have to work so hard to find answers? Why didn't the doctor answer my questions? My sister did not have papers so it was scary to go to the doctor. I was really wanting someone who could help me. Then, I realized that I could be that person, so I went to talk to a college with programs for children with learning disabilities to see if there were free classes. First, I sat in on classes and learned English at Brooklyn Community College. Then, I was able to start studies at La Guardia Community College. That is how I started to do this as a career.

Because of the lack of an obvious career path for becoming a CHW, most slowly became CHWs through a sequence of jobs, with on-the-job-training in skills provided at each step along the way. They started out just wanting to work with people, not necessarily aiming to be a CHW. In this case, recognition that they could truly help their community through their phone calls, conversations, or visits evolved over time, and at some point they fully embraced being a CHW.

> When I was offered the position, I took it because it interested me to try to increase the immunization and well-child visit rates. When I went out to their homes, I realized what parents were dealing with. Missing the appointment wasn't the issue, that was the least of their worries. So, trying to help these families on a day-to-day basis, it became really rewarding to see them take these tiny steps, to be on time for appointments, try to get a better appointment. It just became really rewarding at the time, and it still is.

Who Makes the Best Community Health Worker? Preferred Attributes for Community Health Workers

While a person may be motivated to give back to the community, to help others, that does not mean that he or she is going to have the right combination of personal strengths to be able to work effectively as a CHW. Most reviews of CHW roles have focused on their functional roles, not their attributes, but it is important to recognize that there are qualities which contribute to being a CHW, qualities for which there is no training (Rosenthal, 1998). Those considering becoming a CHW, as well as those who would recruit them for this work, need to know who will make a good CHW.

The most salient characteristic of CHWs is that they be residents of the community where they work (Lehmann and Sanders, 2007). Increasingly, however, the CHW can be recruited from outside the community, as long as the CHW shares a similar culture and life experiences with the community. The loosening of the expectation that the CHW be a resident of the community in which he or she works is important for CHWs promoting the health of immigrants. If the CHW is a fellow immigrant, especially from the country or region from which most in the community come, the CHW will still share critical dimensions of culture and life experiences invaluable to his or her work.

Worldwide, there is a preference for women, who are married and "mature." Since many CHWs work to promote reproductive, maternal, and child health, it is helpful if they are themselves mothers, who will have their own experience to build on when working with community residents. Particularly for CHWs recruited to work in rural communities, it is also felt that married women living in the community will be less likely to abandon their posts to search work in the city. Because CHWs make home visits, whether in New York City or in rural Nicaragua, it is important for those selected to be CHWs be welcome to the homes and, specifically, to interact with women who are the main clients of CHW services in many settings. Women are preferred in this role, not only because of their personal experience with maternal and child health issues but also because their home visits do not arouse suspicions of impropriety. This goes both ways, particularly for immigrant women who fear being sexually exploited by men, even if they appear to be otherwise trustworthy community members. It also has been shown that women are more likely to stay in their posts and are less likely to leave as soon as "better" positions open up elsewhere (Singh and CHW Technical Task Force, 2011).

In contrast to other health workers, most CHW programs in low-income countries do not require secondary education and require only basic literacy or primary school completion. While this may make it more difficult to provide training to the CHW for home-based clinical interventions, it increases the chance of recruitment and retention of CHWs in their communities, as secondary school graduates are more likely to quit their village in pursuit of a job in the city (Lehmann and Sanders, 2007; Tran et al., 2014). In the case of CHWs, too much education may result in a distance between the CHW and the community, which will impede the ability of the CHW to inspire trust or to communicate freely with the community. Educational requirements also could reduce the average age of the CHW, which is at cross purposes with finding people who are experienced and able to command respect from their communities (Lehmann and Sanders, 2007).

Globally, apart from being a member of the community they serve, the most important attribute of the CHW is to be respected, to be considered trustworthy (Tran et al., 2014). Community recruitment is part of the process that communities can use to ensure that the CHWs selected are indeed trustworthy. Without this trustworthiness, the CHW will find it difficult to fully engage the community residents in open discussions about how they might make changes in their lives (Farrar, Morgan, Chuang, and Konrad, 2011; Rosenthal et al., 2010). In multiple studies referenced in Chapter 2, being a fellow immigrant was considered a major door-opener for other immigrants, for whom a fellow immigrant is already one element in the foundation of trust.

Because a large part of the CHW role involves communication, people who are good "communicators" are likely to have success as CHWs (Suter et al., 2009). Along the same lines, the ability to speak the language of the community and understand and demonstrate adherence to the cultural norms will enhance the potential of the CHW to communicate with others (O'Brien, Squires, Bixby, and Larson, 2009). Again, shared language, even down to the local dialect, is essential for the CHWs to serve an immigrant community.

CHWs are expected to be hardworking and responsible. While not all CHWs are peer educators, all are expected to be able to lead by example. They work independently in the community, and they must develop their own routine and activity plan to ensure that they accomplish their responsibilities. The CHW must plan home visits around a multitude of responsibilities, and the weekly or monthly activities must be coordinated with the demands of their own and the work of those they visit (Tran et al., 2014). In the United States, this has often meant that CHWs do a lot of their work in the evenings and weekends. People who are able to manage their time are likely to be more successful CHWs than those who barely manage.

Finally, creativity and resourcefulness are important (Matos, Findley, Hicks, and Do Canto, 2011; Tran et al., 2014). Every CHW has to be able to think on his or her feet, so that the suggestions and support he or she offers to the individual are tailored to that person's specific needs. This requires a certain degree of flexibility and creativity that will allow the CHW to adapt the message as needed or to create novel approaches to helping families make changes.

Refining the Details: What New Yorkers See as Preferred Community Health Worker Attributes

These general characteristics might be ones you would consider appropriate for teachers, nurses, or several other professions, and greater precision is needed if they are to guide people in their choices to become a CHW and also to those wanting to hire people who will make good CHWs. In New York, we went about defining these specific attributes as part of our statewide effort to develop standards for CHWs, their scope of practice, training and certification standards, and financing options. (For details see Matos et al., 2011.) As is the case with members of any other profession establishing standards for itself, CHWs have taken the lead in identifying appropriate attributes for "who" they are, while their employers have tended to focus on "what they do," the roles or activities making up their scope of practice (Catalani, Findley,

Matos, and Rodriguez, 2009). We concluded that if there is to be agreement on scope of practice, it is critical that each group, CHWs and their employers, agree on both the "who" and "what" questions.

To develop a consensus scope of practice for New York, we set out to determine CHWs' perceptions of their attributes (who they are), the roles or the scope of practice they would be expected to fulfill, and skills they considered to be essential for fulfilling these roles. We asked both CHWs and employers to give us their views on all three of these elements, and then we compared the different patterns and distilled out a consensus set of attributes, skills, and roles. (For further details, see Findley et al., 2012.)

We first considered the usual selection criteria for CHWs: that they live in the community where they work. Two thirds of the surveyed CHWs (*n* = 190) lived in or near the community in which they work. As shown in Figure 3.3, three fourths felt it is important to live in or near the community, because it gives them valuable insider knowledge of the community and enables them to understand behaviors of community residents. Just over half of the CHWs surveyed considered community residence important, because it gives them the same frame of reference for modeling behavior change, helps them know organizations where they can make referrals, helps them share values and blend in with residents, and facilitates building trust and rapport.

In contrast to the overwhelming CHW preference for living in or near the community in which they work, only 46% of the employers (*n* = 23) considered residence in the same community important to their decision about who to hire. However, there was agreement by 75% of the employers that CHWs

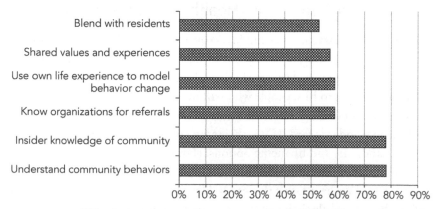

FIGURE 3.3 Why is it important for a community health worker to live in the community?

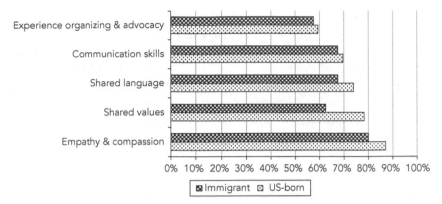

FIGURE 3.4 Most important attribute for a community health worker by community health worker immigrant status, New York CHW Survey 2008–2010.

should have shared values and experiences with residents and that they share the same language as residents with whom they work.

The New York CHWs next rated the general background characteristics, such as language, shared values, or communication. As shown in Figure 3.4 the surveyed CHWs (*n* = 158 with valid responses) said that the most important attribute or general background characteristic was to have empathy and compassion (83%), followed by shared values, shared language, and verbal and nonverbal communication skills. Just over half (58%) considered experience organizing the most important attributed. There was little difference between how US-born and immigrant CHWs rated the attributes, with the exception of shared values, which was less important for the immigrants than for the US-born CHWs.

To further clarify the most desirable attributes for CHWs, further discussion among the participants of the Scope of Practice Working Group of the New York State CHW Initiative yielded the character attributes shown in Table 3.1 as those most highly recommended for CHWs. The attributes recommended by New Yorkers provide important clarifying details to the general list commonly found in national or global standards, and they reflect the context of work in New York, with a very diverse cultural mix of people from many countries, ethnicities, and backgrounds. As can be seen from the attributes, these are personality characteristics that emphasize connection to the community, empathy, openness, and communication, but they also include other qualities that make it possible for the CHW to be creative and find the best ways to support people while juggling different responsibilities.

Table 3.1 CHW Qualities Contributing to Successful Accomplishment of the CHW Scope of Practice

1. Connected to community
   - Community member OR have a close understanding of community
   - Shared life experiences
   - Desires to help the community

2. Empathetic and caring
   - Sensitive
   - Compassionate
   - Considerate
   - Gentle

3. Creative and resourceful
   - Imaginative
   - Ingenious
   - Motivated and capable of self-directed work

4. Open-minded/non-judgmental
   - Unbiased
   - Flexible
   - Tolerant

5. Patient and persistent
   - Prudent
   - Temperate
   - Wise

6. Honest and respectful
   - Sincere
   - Candid
   - Polite
   - Courteous

7. Friendly, outgoing, sociable
   - Responsive
   - Welcoming
   - Pleasant

8. Dependable and reliable
   - Trustworthy
   - Responsible
   - Loyal

When thinking how a CHW will work with immigrants, perhaps the most crucial attributes are the first three: connection to the community, empathy, and creativity. In our in-depth interviews with immigrants ($n = 28$) the single most important criterion that came up repeatedly was that they preferred the CHW to be an immigrant, which means being a member of the immigrant community, whether or not they are also residents of the community where the CHW will be working. Here is what two immigrant CHWs said about the importance of the shared immigrant experience.

> Being that I'm Hispanic and Dominican, that helps me out. I can identify with the problems that a lot of the families are having in the neighborhood.
>
> Through my struggles, my experiences, trying to navigate the system, I had to learn. I was 17 when I came to this country, and I had to mature fast so that I could help others, especially other immigrants. They had the same issues, dreams, and hopes as I had. This is what helped me to choose my career as a CHW.

Among the immigrants who have traversed dangerous times, often alone and in fear of deportation, those who then go on to become CHWs are deeply committed to helping other immigrants obtain documentation and make a life for themselves and their children. Here is Marielena's story of how she transitioned from being alone and homeless to becoming a CHW dedicated to helping other immigrants.

When I first came to this country I was lost and did not have anyone to help me. I had to figure things out for myself. I was illegal and I didn't know anything. It was scary. No one to help me. I didn't know how to navigate the system. I was working in a factory and there was an immigration raid, and I was almost arrested. At that time I thought if I had a passport I was legal, so I didn't know I was illegal. When I realized I was illegal, I left the factory and knew that I needed to do something to get legal in the country. For a while I was homeless and slept on the train. Then I asked a few people how to do it, and they said I should get in a relationship with a man who would sponsor me, so I met someone who I thought would help me, but he wanted to rape me for the favor, so I left. Then I tried another job and became a nanny. Luckily, those people sponsored me so I could become a legal resident. After working for them another 2 years I decided to work at an organization that helped homeless women, like I had been. I thought I should do something for others so they would not go through the same thing I went through. That is when I started working at Goddard–Riverside with the mentally ill and homeless. I saw those men and women going through the same struggle that I went through. My experience helped me to empathize more with the people and forced me to help them so they would not go through the same thing that I had. I had no one to teach me how to do it, but I just kept learning how to work the system so that I could connect them to legal aid to become legal in the country. It was hard to help them with health issues, since they were illegal. I didn't realize it then but that was the first time I worked as a CHW.

For many immigrant CHWs, the commitment is to the larger immigrant community, as their advocate. This connection and the desire to "give back" is a theme that underpins CHW motivation and contributes to their ability to be persistent in the face of adversity, as articulated by these three immigrant CHWs.

My interest was work with the Latino community to help the families that have come from another country, to give them orientation, to advocate for them. To help them reach their goals in this country. To let them know that they have rights to be healthy and take advantage of health services in this country, even when they are immigrants. Health is very important for the human beings.

I grew up in El Salvador during the civil war, and I was always concerned for justice and equality, helping people. My journey and that of my clients is not that different. I relate very deeply to my clients, because we come from a similar background of being poor and immigrant. Thus, I like to share my experience to show that it is possible for everyone to move forward. Helping people navigate through difficulties by sharing my own experience. I let them know what they will experience based on what I have experienced. Then, they really hear me when I explain the "rules" for how to do it.

After I came to the United States, I began helping out at my children's school. I believe that every community member has the responsibility to share their time and resources. If I know about a program, people come to me to learn about it. In this way, I became a negotiator, the voice of other people, who weren't able to help themselves in similar situations. So I was able to become a CHW, and I discovered that it made me happy, to feel good, that I like to help other people, like grandparents, uneducated, and the schools.

Being understanding, caring, and compassionate are also personal resources upon which the CHW draws for working with immigrants.

The work first is about caring for people. I always care for people and identify with their pain. When I moved to New York, I started part time and I didn't even know about African Services Committee until I went there. Then I realized that I could help other Africans through the agency. Being a peer worker, I could work with people. Share with them my experience.

My desire is to help other people. There are a lot of people who need help in different ways. I help them by counseling, helping them to find what they need in the community. Through church, through any agency in the community.

I believe that a great success of these community programs is that they deliver a message for the immigrants telling them: "You are not alone. Even though the system seems to be against you, you can find help and you are not the only one going through these difficult experiences." The health system tells them that they cannot get help because they are undocumented or poor, but we send them a message that there is something to do. Our work promotes solidarity and strengthens the social network among immigrants. They share their own experiences and it builds up community and helps to consolidate the identity of the community.

Being creative and resourceful also is a background characteristic that contributes to CHW success, as in the case of this woman who described how she created a resource book to use when trying to match families with available community resources.

I know where to send families to get help even if they don't have insurance because I have lived here and know the community. I have a resource book that I have made myself. I use it with families in the center, and also with groups in the community. They all know me and from my own experience I know so many places they can go to get help. I know how to help them get help; for example, for boys who are violent or acting out, I tell them about Family Court and Boy's Town in the Bronx. If I don't know, I find out what/ where they can get help, so I can then tell them. I always can find a place or way to help them when they face difficulties.

What Do Community Health Workers Do to Become Influential?

While CHWs may have very different activities and responsibilities, depending on whether they are generalists or specialists focusing on one specific health issue, common to all CHWs are some basic roles, which are associated with core competencies, the skills which all CHWs are expected to have in order to perform their functions. In the United States, the seven basic roles of CHWs were identified in the 1998 National Community Health Advisor Study (Rosenthal, 1998):

- Bridging/cultural mediation between communities and health and social service systems
- Providing culturally appropriate health education and information
- Referring people to the health and social/economic services they need
- Providing informal counseling and social support
- Advocating for individual and community needs
- Providing direct service, such as basic first aid and administering health screening tests
- Building individual and community empowerment capacity

CHWs also play other important roles, which can be considered core competencies:

- Community organizing and advocacy for social justice and equality
- Helping people address broader cultural, environmental, and lifestyle issues that impact health
- Helping patients and community members navigate complex health and social service systems and understand and manage their conditions
- Conducting outreach to isolated or difficult-to-reach populations
- Coordinating care for people with chronic conditions
- Facilitating enrollment in health coverage programs

There is always a tension between not giving the CHWs enough responsibility and overloading the CHWs with too many roles and responsibilities. The trend now is to provide CHWs with core competency training, so they can become "generalist" CHWs, often including skills needed to support community empowerment and advocacy for environmental, social and economic justice, as well as practical skills for helping people with their search for jobs and educational opportunities. In addition, many CHWs are now trained for more specialized tasks of health promotion and adherence coaching, care coordination and case management targeted to specific health issues, such as newborn care, immunization promotion, breastfeeding peer counselors, HIV anti-retroviral medication adherence, diabetes management, or asthma control, to name just a few (Bhutta et al., 2010; Findley et al., 2012; Lehmann and Sanders, 2007; Matos et al., 2011; Tran et al., 2014).

Our experience with the New York State CHW Initiative illustrates the care needed to establish a balance in the scope of practice guidelines between core or basic skills and more advanced skills needed for some but not all CHW positions. Using standardized Internet-based surveys approved by the CUMC IRB, we asked 223 CHWs and 40 employers to rank the most important contributions of CHWs. Half of each group, CHWs and employers, agreed that the following roles were important contributions of the CHWs: making referrals and facilitating access to social services, establishing trust and building rapport between health system and community, providing social support, aiding in patient navigation or escort service, translating and facilitating communication with health care providers, retaining clients, improving health outcomes, visiting homes, providing health education, and performing outreach and enrollment. They also reviewed the specific recommendations from CHWs and employers regarding roles and specific tasks to include in the New York State CHW scope of practice recommendations, and using an iterative process they developed the following scope of practice recommendations regarding the basic roles for NYS CHWs:

> outreach and community mobilization, community/cultural liaison, case management and care coordination, home-based support, health promotion and health coaching, system navigation, and participatory research.

(For details see Findley et al., 2012.)

Table 3.2 shows the similarities in core competency skills obtained from global, US national, and the New York State perspectives. Almost all the core competency skills identified by the New York State group are also considered core skills from the global and national perspectives. The recommendations from the national Community Health Advisor Study do not include training in participatory research and some of the monitoring and data management skills, but this may also be related to the fact that this review was published in 1998, well before computer skills became part of routine documentation now expected of most CHWs globally.

The New York team further clarified the core competencies into major skill categories, as would be used when developing training modules. The 223 CHWs and 40 employers interviewed in the study agreed on the following sets of skills as the basic skill clusters CHWs need.

- *Interpersonal:* Ability to establish trust, bilingual, multicultural competence, providing social support
- *Communication:* Advocacy (individual or community), community organizing, outreach and enrollment, information sharing, listening, goal setting, informal counseling, leading group discussions, facilitating workshops and events, case management and referrals, medical interpretation, interfacing with physicians and health care system

Table 3.2 Comparison of Core Roles by Region, Global, US, and New York

Core Role	Global Health Workforce Alliance (2010) and Tran et al. (2014)	National CHW Study (1998)	NYS CHW Initiative (2012)
Community engagement and bridging between the community and health system	Community engagement and knowledge of community	Bridging and outreach	Community/cultural liaison
Counseling	Counseling	Counseling	Case management and care coordination
Interpersonal communication	Interpersonal communication	Counseling includes communication	Home-based support includes communication
Advocacy	*Not included*	Advocacy	Outreach and community mobilization includes advocacy
Health promotion	Health promotion	Health education	Health promotion and health coaching
Use of behaviour change frameworks	Use behaviour change framework	*Not included*	Health promotion and coaching includes behaviour change
Referrals for health and social services	Identify health conditions and make referrals	Referrals and help getting insurance	Case management and care coordination includes referrals
Information sharing	Appropriate information sharing	Included in translation	Community/cultural liaison includes info exchange
Maintaining privacy and confidentiality	Privacy and confidentiality	*Not included*	Participatory research includes privacy
Organizing, planning, and record keeping	Organization, planning, and record keeping	*Not included*	Documentation and planning in several roles
Participatory research	*Not included*	*Not included*	Participatory research
Teamwork	Teamwork	*Not included*	System navigation and case management and care coordination include teamwork

- *Teaching:* Health education skills, role plays and health behavior modeling, adult learning techniques, chronic disease management supports, home assessment and advice on daily routines, personal safety on home visits
- *Organizational:* Computer skills, time management and scheduling, documentation and data collection, mentoring other CHWs, research procedures

We asked CHWs how they learned these skills, and we were particularly interested in whether the process of learning these skills differed between immigrant and US-born CHWs. Table 3.3 shows for which of the 23 possible skills CHWs ($n = 119$) received training, with the skills for which 50% or more received training highlighted in **bold**.

The CHWs were provided training primarily in communication and teaching skills, with the top five skills for which training was provided being health education (64%), information sharing (59%), data entry and documentation (59%), outreach (56%), and advocacy (56%). Data entry and documentation may seem a nonessential skill, but the CHWs were given training in completing the paperwork they needed to document their work and submit it electronically to their supervisors. Employers' training did not cover several of the organizational skills, and they also omitted explicit training on interpersonal skills.

There were some notable differences in training provided to the immigrants versus the US-born. Within the communications skills group, more immigrants than US-born CHWs received training in the full complement of communication skills, with 60% or more of the immigrants receiving five of the key communication skills training, and 50% or more receiving training in all but one of the communication skills. The immigrant CHWs also were more likely to receive training in the complementary teaching skills of adult learning, goal setting, and adherence promotion, and over half of the immigrant CHWs received training in how to provide social support. Indeed, the only skill on which the US-born received training in greater numbers than among the immigrant CHWs was health education, for which 66% received training. These differences suggest a couple of possible underlying factors: the immigrant CHWs may start out with less experience as CHWs and therefore need more training, they may change jobs more often and receive additional training each time they change jobs, or they may be employed for programs where the objectives are recognized to require a more complete set of skills. Given the challenges of working with immigrants who may be unable or

Table 3.3 Training Received by Skill Set by Community Health Worker Immigration Status, New York Community Health Workers 2010

Skills for Which Received Training	Total	US-born	Immigrant
Interpersonal and organizing			
Establish trust	10%	7%	15%
Outreach	**56%**	**56%**	**56%**
Bilingual	30%	27%	35%
Multicultural competence	39%	38%	42%
Social support	47%	44%	**52%**
Communications			
Workshop organization	**55%**	**51%**	**63%**
Advocacy	**56%**	**53%**	**62%**
Information sharing	**59%**	**57%**	**62%**
Group discussions	46%	43%	**53%**
Lead group events	**51%**	45%	**64%**
Listening	**54%**	**50%**	**63%**
Informal counseling	33%	28%	45%
Case management	**53%**	**52%**	**56%**
Teaching			
Health education	**64%**	**66%**	**59%**
Adult learning	46%	43%	**51%**
Goal setting	**54%**	**51%**	**59%**
Adherence promotion	48%	43%	**57%**
Home assessment and tailoring daily routine	36%	36%	35%
Personal safety	35%	36%	33%
Organizational			
Medical interpretation	48%	**51%**	41%
Patient navigation	45%	45%	44%
Time management	48%	44%	**55%**
Research	27%	26%	30%
Mentoring other community health workers	38%	36%	43%
Supervisory skills	33%	35%	28%
Data entry and documentation	**59%**	**55%**	**68%**
Computer skills	44%	42%	49%

Note: Skills for which 50% or more received training highlighted in **bold**.

unwilling to access health services, it is likely that the latter may play an important role in the provision of training for the immigrant CHWs.

Which of these skills were actually used by the CHWs? Three fourths or more of the CHWs reported using all the interpersonal, communication, and teaching skills, with the exception of mentoring, medical interpretation, home assessment, and patient navigation, which were used by 60%–74% of the CHWs. All communication skills except adult learning were used by 100% of the CHWs, as were three organizational skills: computer use, time management, and workshop organizing. The only skills used by fewer than 60% of the CHWs were the supervisory and research skills.

When actually doing their work, people do not analyze what they do, skill by skill or task by task, so it is hard to capture which of the skills has the most influence. When asked about the most critical elements of their work, without which the other elements will not work, CHWs commented repeatedly on the importance of building a trusting relation and face-to-face meetings outside of the health system, a "comfortable place where their privacy is respected so people feel free to come."

> The first step I would recommend is to know the culture. Having a phone will help also so that the immigrants can get used to talking about their health problems, even if not yet face to face. You have to convey confidentiality and privacy, so they feel safe and trust you. Then you can talk face to face. The immigrants want to be sure that their culture is respected as they go from test to test, doctor to doctor, within the health system.

Not all CHW programs include making home visits, but according to the CHW feedback, these are very important for establishing a trusting relation and then being able to work together constructively. These personalized visits play a key role in establishing the trust needed between the CHWs and immigrants, particularly given the precarious situation of many immigrants with whom they work. This CHW who works with immigrant families to promote childhood immunizations aptly captured the essence of this relation:

> So I think the hardest thing in educating these older parents is they have a mindset that they don't deserve better. It goes a little deeper than just the appointment, but I use the appointment and the information that I give them as a hook, to boost their morale a little bit. They just tend to feel that

that's how they are, and that's all they can achieve. So that's a big obstacle. I have to be persistent. I tend to call the resistant parents more often, and usually I go to their home. When we are on their home turf, they feel a little bit more comfortable, and they'll open up a little bit more. So, I try to hang on to them as long as I can, if they're noncompliant, because I think persistence makes them feel more important. Just constant talking, like how are you, what's going on, and what's new, just trying to get them to open up. It's so important in their home, I think, where you can build more of a personal relationship with them.

We hear from a hospital-based CHW about the importance of home visits:

I have to say, I know there's a lot of CHWs who do work from offices, but I think there's a lot of families out there who need the information brought to them, so you can sit down with them and walk them through certain processes. The hospital—speaking from where I work—I know that the clinic discharges clients if they miss numerous appointments. But those people, they have other issues than just missing appointments. They are the neglected ones. So, I feel that we should be reaching out to those families more on their level, going to their homes and trying to actually find out what's going on. We can let them know what's available, because they really won't know unless they come in and get the information. Since they don't, it's not available to them.

Another immigrant CHW working with South Asian immigrant families stressed the importance of repeated home visits.

To do more home visits would reach more immigrants than currently, because sometimes, the people have issues and they don't know how to express the issue when they see you at the office. Even if it's not the first visit, but the second or the third time, they open to you, they express the necessities that they have, and you can help them in a lot of ways.

The employers of the CHWs did not always see the required skill sets and activities with the same priorities as the CHWs. As shown in Figure 3.5, employers agreed with the CHWs that it was most important for the CHW

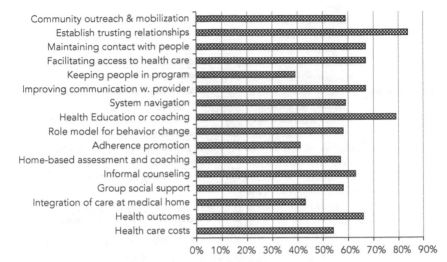

0% 10% 20% 30% 40% 50% 60% 70% 80% 90%

FIGURE 3.5 Importance of community health worker skills to their program, New York CHW Survey 2010.

to establish a trusting relation with the community (84%), although they did not provide training in this. Compared to CHW priorities, they placed more value on CHW educating and coaching (79%) and on facilitating improved communications between the patient and provider (67%). Two thirds of the employers also indicated that the CHWs were appreciated by the program for facilitating community access to health insurance and health care services, maintaining contact with patients, and their contribution to health outcomes. These were less highly ranked by the CHWs, among whom 50%–60% indicated that their program valued their outreach, communication, and organizing skills.

The only skills not highly valued by the program managers were CHW efforts to keep people in the program, adherence promotion, and working within an integrated medical team. These areas also turn up as difficulties experienced by the CHWs, particularly the immigrant CHWs (see Fig. 3.6). Lack of appreciation for their work to keep people in the program comes through in the difficulty that one third of the CHWs find in working simply as "quota-based" enrollers, where the difficulties of recruitment are not appreciated. Related to this is the CHW perception that they do not get enough supportive supervision, which feels more like "bean counting" than constructive suggestions, a difficulty articulated by immigrant CHWs more than US-born CHWs. One third of the immigrant CHWs found lack of integration into the medical team to be a great difficulty. Without being a part of the team,

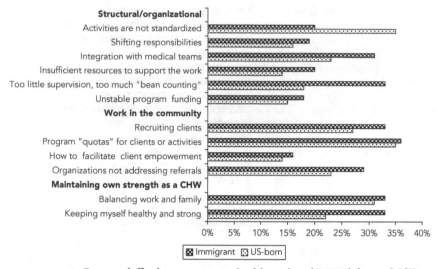

FIGURE 3.6 Greatest difficulties community health workers (CHWs) face in fulfilling their responsibilities by CHW immigrant status, New York CHW Survey 2010.

it was very difficult for the CHWs to perform the bridging function, linking people to health care providers and vice versa.

Being a bridge between the community and the health system is clearly wearing on the CHW, as one third of the CHWs (more immigrant than US-born) found it difficult to maintain personal and professional boundaries, a balance between their work and their own life, and to keep themselves healthy and stress-free. As several of the CHWs noted in their interviews, they want to be available to clients when they need them, but it is difficult to know when to shut off the phone and ignore what could be a call from a person with whom you have worked hard to build a trusting relation. Related to this dilemma is the feeling that they do not know as much as they would like to support empowerment of the client, as well as the perception that the organizations they work with may not be listening, as they do not address all the referrals they make, particularly by the immigrant CHWs.

In the interviews, CHWs raised some of these same issues about the challenges of their work: not enough resources to help everyone in need, too much paperwork, too many meetings; management issues, supervisors task oriented and not people oriented, needing to teach oneself to shut down when leaving work.

Several CHWs recommended a stronger integration of the CHW into the health care team, as this would give CHWs credibility among immigrants that they have a place in the system and can then help them navigate it. Meeting at the facility would position the CHW to be able to help families directly.

> CHWs maybe can start to be in every facility and be there to give advice to the immigrant families, especially the undocumented. You can say, "Let's start with a screening, find out if you are healthy." If we had CHWs everywhere, this would be a big help for the immigrant community. I think it should be more of a team, having a CHW along with a provider, a nurse, a social worker. I think we have to have more friendly, gentle staff who can help the family when they come to the clinic or doctor. To be more helpful for them, not to make it so complicated. Sometimes the clinic puts difficulties for the family, and it should be easier for them to go with the children.

A difficulty that uniquely affects immigrant CHWs is their own immigration status. As we have seen, immigrants who have successfully overcome the myriad of difficulties of getting settled and organizing their lives and health care are keen to help others along the way. Yet those who have experienced the greatest difficulties may still be undocumented, which poses difficulties for them in finding work as CHWs, because employers will have difficulty hiring them. As described previously by Arelia, those who do have valid working papers may still face challenging renewals every year. Ironically, keeping their own job as a CHW becomes a major difficulty, as related by José from Chicago.

> A problem I faced is that I needed to leave my job because my work permit expired and the organization I work with was reluctant to hire me without a permit for a longer period of time. Nor would they sponsor me. Documentation barriers can be a big obstacle to serve the community. I know many immigrants who want to become CHWs, but they cannot because nobody can hire them as undocumented immigrants.

Which Health Problem Areas Do Community Health Workers Work on?

Although over the course of their work life, many CHWs become generalists, most find positions in programs that are focusing on one or more health

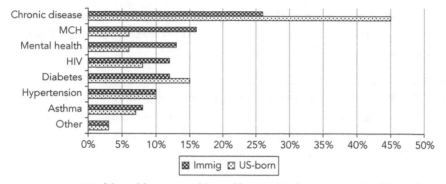

FIGURE 3.7 Health problem areas addressed by New York community health workers by immigrant status, New York CHW Survey 2010.

problem area. The CHW may address multiple related health concerns, such as wellness, diabetes, hypertension, and nutrition or maternal and child health and family planning and reproductive health. Figure 3.7 shows the health problem areas that the New York CHWs covered in their current work or what they had previously addressed, contrasting the areas worked by CHW immigrant status. This figure shows that the New York CHWs are working in most of the health problem areas where CHWs are effective according to our summary in Chapter 2, the areas where there is potential for them to be effective, with the largest concentrations in chronic disease prevention or management, along with very specific programs for prevention and/or control of diabetes, hypertension, and asthma. More of the US-born CHWs (78%) work in these areas than immigrant CHWs (54%). Almost twice as many US-born are working in generalized chronic disease prevention or management programs than immigrant CHWs, 45% versus 26%, and they also are more likely to be working in programs focusing only on diabetes prevention and/or control, 15% versus 12%. Among both groups, 10% are working in programs focused only on hypertension or cardiovascular health, and roughly equivalent shares are working to promote asthma self-management. In contrast, twice as many immigrant CHWs are involved in programs working with women, promoting maternal or child health. They are also twice as likely to be working with immigrants on issues pertaining to mental health, including substance abuse, and more immigrant than US-born CHWs are working in HIV prevention or adherence promotion programs.

Thus, there appears to be selective exclusion of the immigrant CHWs from the areas of chronic disease prevention and management. Yet these are precisely the areas where immigrants most need help, and for which there is substantial evidence of their effectiveness. While the immigrant CHWs can certainly assist with the more episodic care issues, as those related to pregnancy and child birth, there is clearly a need for programs working with chronic disease prevention and management to reach out and include more immigrants among the CHWs they train and hire for this work.

How Do Their Clients Recognize the Community Health Worker's Influence?

Which activities were most appreciated by the people with whom the CHWs work? It is not possible for CHWs to ask about feedback about each of their 20+ activities, but the CHWs were able to indicate which general activities were most appreciated. As shown in Figure 3.8, regardless of their place of birth, 84% of the CHWs reported that people most appreciated their efforts to establish a trusting relation, followed by improved health outcomes, for which the immigrant CHWs reported much higher approval ratings than the US-born CHWs, and health education and coaching, for which the US-born immigrants reported greater appreciation than immigrant CHWs. While both groups reported high approval from program participants for the CHW's help in staying in contact with the program, they differed slightly in the relative appreciation for their help in gaining access to health care (more positive for the US-born CHWs) and in what they got out of informal

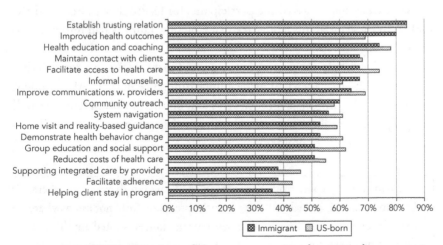

FIGURE 3.8 CHW perceptions of their most appreciated activities by community health worker immigration status, New York CHW Survey 2010.

counseling (more positive for the immigrant CHWs). While it would have been expected that the immigrant CHWs would be more valuable in improving communication with providers and in system navigation, the US-born CHWs appear to have been more greatly appreciated for these efforts.

These differences in valuation of their work underscore the importance that CHWs be equipped at a minimum with the skills most valued by their clients. CHWs need feedback on what is really making a difference to the clients, so that they can tailor their efforts accordingly.

Community Health Worker Influence: Feedback From Immigrants on Community Health Worker Influence

Over the last 15 years, we have also been able to obtain feedback from participants on the contributions of the CHWs. These programs have included the New York State Department of Health's support for CHWs in federal/state funded parenting support programs (Healthy Families USA and Healthy Start) as well as several programs under the umbrella of the Northern Manhattan Community Voices initiative (to be discussed in greater depth in the next chapter). Across all these programs we asked participants to anonymously tell us what they liked most and liked least about their programs, as well as to give specific feedback on the CHWs with whom they worked. For this chapter, we reviewed the feedback responses from 254 individuals, mostly women, who had participated in these programs between 1998 and 2012. At the same time that we asked the participants for feedback, we also asked 102 CHWs in these programs to give feedback on how families had responded to their efforts.

Overwhelmingly, the participants reported that CHWs had done all that they could, and that they had made a huge difference in their lives. Namely, CHWs had a big influence on their lives and on their health. Here is a small sampling of the feedback we received from participants working with CHWs across a wide variety of programs.

> I had recently come from Barbados, and all my family was back there. I was living alone, and when I was 5 months pregnant, I did not know where to go for prenatal care. The father of the baby no longer wanted anything to do with me. I was unemployed and did not have money. I did not have the proper immigration papers, so I did not think I could qualify for any health

care. So I went to CAMBA [a well-known community organization support-ing Caribbean immigrants, near her home]. The CHW explained that I was eligible for New York's program of assistance to pregnant and newborns, the PCAP program [now MOMS], as well as for WIC. She enrolled me in both programs and gave me valuable nutritional and developmental infor-mation about my pregnancy. The CHW also helped me with my financial difficulties. I had been receiving help from my father with monthly expenses, but he had recently passed away, and now I was 4 months in arrears. When I received the eviction notice, the CHW helped me go through the court process and this kept me from getting evicted. The CHW also helped me when my baby was born. The baby was born premature and had to be kept in the hospital NICU for 2 weeks after I was discharged. The CHW often accompanied me to the hospital and helped me bond with my baby. She advocated with the hospital to get me a breast pump so that my daughter could receive breast milk while she was in the NICU. Thus, when the baby came home, I was able to continue breastfeeding, and now I have a thriving 4-month old, all thanks to my CHW at CAMBA.

I was depressed and isolated; most of my friends were having fun but I was too sick. When I first came to the program, I did not want to be there and thought I would drop out. But with time I saw what other people were doing, so I started accepting it and participating. With the help of the nutri-tion class, I take better care of myself. I feel better now, because I can control more what I eat. I feel motivated. I want to learn more. I know that the only one that's really going to benefit from the changes will be me. The program does not need any changes to make it better. We are the ones who need to make changes, taking advantage of what you teach.

This is a poor neighborhood, and someone has to take charge and help out the poor. Alianza is doing it. This is an office that helps the commu-nity so much, so much, so much. I am so thankful to them. The people are very kind. There are a lot of Dominican people there. They help you out a lot. Anyone I know that comes and has problems with rent, or the court, or whatever, I say to them, "Let's go to Alianza so they can help you." Many people that live in the neighborhood don't know what there is available for them. It satisfies me that a friend will tell me that she got whatever she needed taken care of when she saw the people [the CHWs] at Alianza.

I was very depressed. I used to be addicted to bananas. I would buy a whole stalk of bananas, and then eat them as they got ripe. Every day, I would have two bananas with my coffee, six cups with sugar. Letty [my CHW] suggested that bananas and coffee with sugar both have a lot of sugar, and advised me to cut back little by little. She motivated me. So, I tried it, cutting back first on the sugar in my coffee. That was my first small step. Then after the next visit, I started cutting back on both bananas and coffee, little by little. So now, my coffee is without sugar and no more bananas. My life changed because of her visits. Before, I couldn't come to the group, because I was too tired and could not walk. But after I stopped eating all the bananas, I started coming to the group. Now I come every week. I am happy and proud to be working on my problems.

In addition to providing feedback directly to the program evaluation team, the program participants have many ways of letting the CHW know about their influence. Just as the CHWs learn to use appropriate body language and non-verbal communication to listen to and support their clients, the clients in turn relay their appreciation for the CHW using smiles and their friendly, welcoming demeanor when they interact with the CHWs. Many CHWs commented on how pleased they were to see their clients smile. Indeed, the nonverbal cues are a sign that rapport has been established between the CHW and the client.

I was just starting to work with a woman who had diabetes, income problems, depression, so I expected this to be a difficult case. But, when I went to her house, it was magical. I could not teach this. When I approached her, she felt that comfortable with my presence. At the beginning she was very serious, closed, but by the end she was smiling. We established rapport during this one visit.

Beyond the nonverbal cues, many participants thanked the CHW directly for the help they received and the impact it made on their lives. They are grateful to learn to do things themselves and to get ahead, as relayed by two CHWs we interviewed.

Sometimes somebody will call to thank me for my help. They say, "You were there for me, you helped me. I called you even late at night and you were there for me." This is enough for me to know that I helped them to know the system and that they survived. When I meet others I have worked with who have a successful life- went to school, got a job- this is also rewarding to me. They came with nothing and then they got jobs, work in a restaurant, a taxi to drive, and work, work, work. Then, they eventually go to school at the same time. A lot of them really succeed in this country.

I love my community. I love doing my job. Not because of my pay—I could go to a provider and get $35,000–$45,000, but I like seeing the smile on someone's face and hearing a thank-you. That means more than another zero on my paycheck.

Another way that the CHWs see the influence they have on others is through people's interactions among themselves and their individual development and empowerment. In many programs CHWs provide social support and coaching through both individual and group sessions. The group sessions are partially educational, usually focusing on one topic per session, but more important participants can explain how they have made changes and encourage others to follow in their footsteps, as a CHW at Alianza told us.

People are comfortable coming to a place they know. People feel comfortable here at Alianza. They can share, they can be open about what they eat; there are no barriers in expressing themselves. They can be honest about their issues. They can talk to each other, help each other, share their perspectives on what they observe or experience. This helps to spread things among the group. They see how others have changed, and then they see what they have to change. This helps break the pattern, helping people change habits. It would not be the same at a clinic, even if we were the same people. The hospital constrains people. They are afraid to express themselves to doctors and nurses [for fear of being judged and punished]. What do we do that is different is that the change happens here among each other, and not with the doctor: They can start here little by little, step by step. When they hear from other participants, they can see that other people are also able to make changes.

This last comment is particularly powerful in that it highlights the vitality and enormously empowering effect of the shared-power relationship CHWs have with the people they serve. As the CHWs observe the changes happening among the people with whom they work, it is doubly rewarding—to the individuals making the change and to the CHW who knows he or she has contributed to helping this change happen.

I feel great when the client has one of those "light bulb" moments, when they connect what they have been learning from me and what is going on in their family. Seeing things fall into place for clients after working with the various providers to meet her needs is very rewarding.

It is very rewarding when I see any little change in a woman with a lot of problems, when they start meeting their goals. I recall one client. She was pregnant and using drugs when she came into the program, and now she is no longer using drugs, has a healthy baby, and is seeing a nutritionist as part of a weight loss program. I love seeing them grow and learn so they don't even need me anymore.

In the program where I work now, I spend 5 years with a family, and this is long enough to see differences being made. I can see mothers enrolling in WIC, learning English, taking part in job training programs, getting jobs. These achievements are very rewarding.

You can see the growth throughout the years, when they have another child who drops into my lap in the system again. I can see the differences, compared to what they learned with the first child. They achieved more, they feel better about themselves. This means they're more responsible for the child's health, and I think that's really great to see when you have a family or a young mom with multiple children, to see the difference from one child to the next, once you help them feel better about themselves.

Beyond observing these changes, occasionally, the impact of the CHW is literally lifesaving or hugely transforming, immediately visible to the CHW and the client's family. While such events may—be rare, what is remarkable about them is that they show the importance of the CHW being present, being there for the family when they urgently need help. We return again to Karime to hear his story of how a simple phone call made all the difference in the world.

There was a woman in labor at a hospital in the Bronx, and she needed a Caesarean-section. The doctors were all ready, but they were unable to convince the husband to give his permission. Even though the life of the woman was on the line, he did not agree. He was scared that she would die with the surgery. He also believed that what was going to happen was the will of God, so [he believed] they should not intervene. The doctors knew about the work of African Services Committee, so they paged me to come to the hospital to talk with the couple in their own language. When I arrived, I greeted the husband with the respectful Muslim greeting, "A Salaam Alekkum," and that told the husband right away that I was a believer. Having gained his trust, I was then able to explain that the procedure also was coming from God, with the doctor doing it. The way that I approached him he was able to understand the problem and what needed to be done. I was able to explain that the lives of the mother and baby could be saved. So, the husband gave permission and the surgery was performed. The hospital had all the technology it needed, but did not have the human resources to use them. This showed the importance of the CHW to ensure that the hospital could do its job. Without my presence, she would have died.

Usually, however, change is slow. The CHWs know they are not miracle workers. This is hard work, and the CHW knows the mantra of step by step, little by little, as described earlier. This work requires patience, as change does not happen overnight. Here are three accounts from CHWs of their proudest moments:

My greatest satisfaction is to make an impact on people's lives. The impact of a CHW is on their knowledge, their lives, and then on their health. Changing habits is a process, too. When people come here to the nutrition class, they are used to eating white rice. They say that is the way my mother did it for me, and that is what I am doing. But, when they start the class, they taste the brown rice, and they like it. Then, they learn how to cook it, and in this way they are able to change their habit of eating white rice. Little by little, you can make a change in people's way of doing things. The CHW can do that by being patient and working with people. Once they have started to make one change to their habits, it is then easier to help them with other habits.

I remember a young lady on public assistance, who was a caregiver for her mother, also on public assistance. Her mother was very sick with asthma and had many doctor's visits and needed much care. Her daughter, Maria, had never worked, and she was bitter and angry at her mother. They were both very unhappy with their life situations and had lost any compassion or support for each other. After working with me in support of her mother, Maria confessed that she wanted to work outside the house, but she had no confidence and did not know what she could do. I worked with her to help her find her strengths, and she saw that she was very organized (getting mom to appointments on time), could keep records (kept track of meds), and she was articulate with a good phone voice. So, after this discussion, I helped Maria create a resume, which she then marketed and got a job. It was very moving for me to be in that role. I did nothing except help her realize her capacities. In our world, usually there is no space for that kind of discussion. I remember clearly when she got the job and what a difference it made in her life: She got off welfare, went back to school. You get to do this when you are a CHW. Not all jobs let you do that.

Two things are my greatest accomplishments: I have been able to ease suffering, broadly, not just in health. Helping people become comfortable and confident in accessing services. Helping them to overcome myths and legends, fear of government, police, expenses. In many countries if you use social services it counts against you socially, so they have fears of using social services because it might impact their visa application or residency. It is horrible to be afraid of every authoritative figure and the police. My other big accomplishment is to help people realize their strengths and abilities. I help them package that into a marketable asset. I help them see that their abilities make them employable. I help them make a resume out of these qualities. This is empowerment. When otherwise they don't feel they can make a contribution, it builds individual capacity, strengthens families and communities.

Immigrant CHWs often help other immigrants in overcoming the same barriers they encountered when they were newly immigrated, opening doors for their clients to get emergency health insurance, find housing, enroll in educational or social service programs, and to obtain referrals to legal assistance for immigration documents. They use their personal experience in overcoming adversity as a guide and motivator for their clients. Two CHWs working with a community Head Start program shared how they work with other immigrants.

I often share my own experience, that I also had difficulties and had to overcome them. I want to make sure that people know we can use programs, even though we come from another country. When I tell them about me, they understand that they can have benefits here. I help them get insurance, so they can go to the doctor.

I know where to send families to get help even if they don't have insurance, because I have lived here and know the community. I have a resource book that I have made myself. I use it with families in the center, and also with groups in the community. They all know me and from my own experience I know so many places they can go to help. If I don't know, I find out what and where they can get help, so I can then tell them. I think I have been successful in helping families get health care when they don't have insurance. I take them, spend the whole day so that they know how and where to go to the doctor, how to get medicines. Afterward, I feel so good, because then the family has good health, and they can continue fighting for the family. I had one family that was like a little tree dying, but then I helped her with her kids, and now she is going along and able to do so many things for herself.

Immigrant CHWs also promote networking, to help the new immigrants forge connections, so they are not alone, as described by a CHW we have already heard from before, whose message is so pertinent to the importance of building personal networks.

I believe that a great success of these community programs is that they deliver a message for the immigrants telling them: "You are not alone. Even though the system seems to be against you, you can find help and you are not the only one going through these difficult experiences." The health system tells them that they cannot get help because they are undocumented or poor, but we send them a message that there is something they can do. Our work promotes solidarity and strengthens the social network among immigrants.

The last story in this chapter is from a young Moroccan immigrant in Montreal, Canada, who has worked as a CHW with immigrant families experiencing asthma and other chronic health problems. With the advantage of working in Canada, where the health care system does not create barriers between immigrants and health insurance that it does in the United States, Fatima's lengthy and eloquent testament shows key processes by which immigrant CHWs become influential with other immigrant families.

I am Muslim, and after September 11, the world changed a lot for Arabic and Muslim people. Here in Canada, discrimination increased after the Commission of Immigrants was established. Because I am an immigrant myself, and I know what it is to be an immigrant arriving in an entirely new country, I have always thought about immigrants' life in the face of this discrimination, and I feel compelled to help the new immigrants

If life is difficult when you are healthy, can you imagine how it is if you are a sick person? Immigrants are very vulnerable, and the health system is very complex in this country. I work as a liaison between the immigrants and organizations that can help them, including medical providers. I also help the medical professionals understand the immigrants they serve. Immigrants come from different cultures, languages, and religions. Sometimes providers ignore the complexity of the problems that immigrants have to face. Health care professionals have to understand these populations. Because some doctors and other health care providers do not know how or where to learn about these important issues that determine immigrants' health, I steer them in the right direction to learn. Immigrants do not like to talk about problems; they do not speak out about their complaints, so we have to help them to be confident enough to speak. Latin American refugees, for example, as well as other undocumented persons, are usually only concerned with survival. They do not ask, or are afraid to ask, for changes in their living conditions even if they are bad for their health. So, with my immigrant background, I can bring all those issues to the doctors' offices and organizations working to improve immigrant's health.

One example is the work I do with environmental health, especially indoor air pollution. Immigrants cannot see the link between their living conditions and their illnesses. In this city, 65% of apartments with indoor air pollution problems are occupied by immigrants, and asthma is a big problem for immigrant children. I help immigrants understand the problem. Another example is how to cope with the cold winters. Immigrants do not know how to live in an apartment in winter. They do not know how to use windows and heaters. So, I help them learn how to live healthy in their apartments. I have to be practical.

My work is very important for immigrants. We help them learn how to live in a new country. Immigrants need a lot of support. They need not only a job, but many other skills to be able to have a quality life in a new setting. They need guidance on many other issues. I can give them that guidance, because it is easy for immigrant women to talk to me. They won't talk openly with anybody else, but with a person like them who speaks their language, they feel confident to express their needs and concerns. For example, I realized that the messages they heard about cooking and measuring food were not easy for them to understand. Some recipes talk about measuring food in cups, but African people use their hands to measure food, not cups. So, if you do not adapt everything to the language that they can understand, the message won't be useful to them. So, I teach them how to measure food.

> After that, we have been successful in improving immigrants' nutrition prac-
> tices. To give another example, people agree that immigrants need spiritual
> care as part of their health. However, in Quebec the majority of services are
> suited for Catholics, not for immigrants who practice other religions. This
> meant that we have had to create more spaces for immigrants to worship and
> receive the spiritual care they need.

In this one statement, Fatima summarizes why she became a CHW. She uses
her immigrant experience to build a trusting relation with the immigrant
women she serves. She also works within the home setting to help immigrants make the small but critical and sustainable changes to their daily lives
that prevent minor health issues from becoming urgent and difficult-to-treat
critical episodes that further challenge their efforts to improve their lives.
Furthermore, she bridges the gap between the doctors and the immigrants,
helping them to have a common understanding and communicate with each
other. The bridge that Fatima builds between immigrants and health care
providers has two-way traffic. She helps the immigrants approach and speak
with the health care provider at the same time that she facilitates the provider's shift in perspective, allowing them to cross that bridge and communicate with their patients with a better understanding of how to help them stay
healthy. With this two-way bridge Fatima's influence goes beyond the direct
impact of her visits to the immigrant's home to a lasting impact on the relation between the immigrant and his or her health care providers. When other
immigrants come to see these providers, the doctor will already have crossed
the bridge before, and it will be that much easier for the next immigrants who
come to their consultation rooms.

Conclusions: Immigrants Becoming Community Health Workers

The journey traversed by men and women who immigrate and then become
CHWs is long and challenging. They have undergone suffering before, during, and after their immigration to their new home. Progress along the way is
marked by the very attributes that go into becoming a successful CHW: courage, perseverance, creativity, flexibility, humanity, and a tenacious determination to making life better for themselves and their families. In the different
ways that they have shared these stories and self-reflections, we see that it
is not by chance that they have become CHWs. This commitment to help

others, to "give back," is salient for all CHWs, but we see it very strongly among the immigrant CHWs. From intention to realization of the CHW dream is another journey in itself, as these immigrants find jobs and learn the dozens of skills they need to become effective and influential as CHWs. Regardless of their immigrant status, CHWs need interpersonal communication, teaching, organizational, and management skills in order to function effectively across the multitude of tasks they are asked to do. When they are able to put all these things together in their work with other immigrants, they are handsomely repaid by the appreciation they receive from their employers and from the people with whom they work. They have influence, and they and everyone they work with can see this.

What are the particular challenges and strategies distinguishing the CHWs who work with immigrants from those who work with the native-born?

- *Shared immigrant background:* These few words embody a host of strengths that the immigrant CHWs bring to their work: compassion, endurance, perseverance, empathy, and understanding of what it means to suffer, to be excluded, and to be able to conquer difficulties, both small and large. In addition to the background, the sharing part is invaluable, as they are able to work within the immigrant community, both in their homes and in groups.
- *Commitment to the immigrant community:* Immigrant CHWs are committed to helping their fellow immigrants, and they are well positioned to become leaders. They use this commitment in their outreach and encouragement to others to get involved in improving health, and it also supports them in being skilled facilitators of the social support groups that are a part of their work. Strongly committed to the welfare and rights of immigrants, the immigrant CHWs also become advocates for immigrant rights, often becoming leaders of immigrant associations. This additional advocacy further supports their work, promoting access to housing, schools, and jobs, so critical to immigrant welfare and their successful impact on individual immigrants in their CHW capacity.
- *Creativity and resourcefulness:* Among the attributes of successful CHWs are being creative and resourceful. In a society where so many of the pathways to success are partially or fully barred to immigrants, the CHW has to be creative and resourceful, to find alternative solutions to problems, to make the proverbial lemonade out of lemons. Fatima's explanation of

translating "cups" into African handfuls is symbolic of the many ways that immigrants translate not just the words but the meanings into concepts that fit within the culture of the immigrant and allow the immigrants to take steps forward in addressing their problems, whether it is in mastery of healthy recipes or learning the difference between two kinds of medications. Even the barrier of restricted access to health insurance has been one that the immigrant CHWs have helped immigrants overcome, for example by explaining access to which they are entitled, including emergency Medicaid.

- *Interpersonal communication and coaching:* Their communication skills go far beyond simple language translation to enabling cross-cultural communication and understanding between the patient and the provider. In their own lives, they used their strong interpersonal skills, seeking out jobs and housing through their family and community networks, and they have used these communication skills to help other immigrants better navigate interactions with the system. With their training on coaching, they have helped immigrants understand the root causes of their conditions and the health providers' recommendations and translate them into concepts they can understand and implement.
- *Home visits:* In a society where immigrants are fearful of the system and the potential for "the system" to trap and then deport them or to otherwise deny them access to treasured goals, such as family reunification, immigrants are loathe to come to the hospital or clinic unless they have no choice. Strangers who are not immigrants would be equally distrusted in their homes, but the immigrant CHWs are more likely to be welcomed and trusted in the home. Hence, home visits are an essential part of the work that immigrant CHWs do with immigrants.
- *Two-way bridge:* Immigrant CHWs understand that the links they make to the health care system cannot be one-way. While it is important for them to serve as translators and to help immigrants navigate the system, they also see that the immigrants will not fully use this system if they feel unwelcome and misunderstood. Therefore, the bridge that immigrant CHWs build is bidirectional, bringing greater multicultural sensibilities to health care providers and the larger health care system. They have sometimes encountered resistance from the health care system in fully incorporating their input and participation into the health care team, but these failures have not prevented immigrant CHWs from persisting in their efforts to make the bridge two-way.

Perhaps the most powerful lesson in these stories is that the CHW experience is so much more than a job. It is apparent from the stories documented here that CHWs possess an insatiable determination to support human dignity and social justice. The struggles related by the CHWs show that their influence and success with people, and particularly with immigrants, does not result only from the work that they do as individual CHWs with individual immigrants. This is most apparent when we consider the bridge built between the immigrant and the health care system. The very nature of that bridge depends on the community and systems being linked. Building the bridge involves supportive foundations from the community and its collaborating organizations, on one side, and health care providers, on the other. In the next chapter we will broaden our perspective to this wider community, seeing how CHWs work within systems and communities and over time to build the bridges and facilitate the flows back and forth between community and health system.

4

Community Health Workers Promoting Immigrant Health

HOW COMMUNITY HEALTH WORKERS HAVE SUPPORTED DOMINICAN IMMIGRANTS IN WASHINGTON HEIGHTS, NEW YORK

IN OUR JOURNEY to understand how community health workers (CHWs) are uniquely situated to promote the health of immigrants, it is now time to explore in depth the experiences of one set of programs that work in the context of a specific immigrant community. In this chapter, we focus on our experience working with community coalitions to promote the health of immigrants to New York City, where we live and work. After a brief introduction describing immigrant health issues in New York City, we narrow the focus to Dominicans, one of the top three immigrant groups in the city. Dominicans are concentrated in the Northern Manhattan community of Washington Heights, and the rest of the chapter focuses on the health needs of this community and how several community coalitions incorporated CHWs effectively to reduce chronic disease risk.

New York City: A City of Immigrants

New York City continues to be a major attraction for immigrants to the United States. While vast numbers of immigrants pass through New York City on their way to other destinations, millions have made New York City their home. In 2011, 37.2% of the city's population of 8.2 million was foreign-born. One in thirteen (7.6%) of all immigrants to the United States live in New York City, and the city has a higher density of foreign-born than any other city in the United States. Over half of all the immigrants to New York are from Latin America (32.1%) or Asia (27.5%), with the remainder from the Caribbean (19.4%), Europe (15.9%), Africa (4.2%), and other countries (0.9%). The top three countries of origin for immigrants to New York were the Dominican Republic (380,200), China (350,000), and Mexico (186,300). Just over 1 million of the immigrants arrived in the past decade, from 2000 to 2011. These newcomers now comprise over one third of all foreign-born in the city. The past decade also saw large increases in new immigrants from Bangladesh and Ecuador. By 2011, New York City was home to 54% of all US immigrants from Guyana, 42% from the Dominican Republic, 40% from Bangladesh, 38% from Trinidad and Tobago, and 32% from Ecuador (Lobo and Salvo, 2013).

The immigrants do not settle evenly throughout the city (see Fig. 4.1). Like immigrants everywhere, they settle in neighborhoods where they can find housing and jobs through friends and family who have preceded them, if not from the same city or village, at least from the same country. There are seven neighborhoods that together are home for 474,100 immigrants, larger than the population of the state of Connecticut. For decades, Dominicans have settled in the Manhattan neighborhood of Washington Heights, and they continue to settle there, along with spread into neighboring sections of Upper Manhattan and the Bronx. Upper Manhattan also has become a destination for Central American immigrants. Several neighborhoods in the borough of Queens have become home for many Asian immigrants, along with those

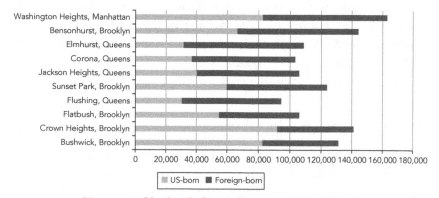

FIGURE 4.1 Top 10 neighborhoods for immigrants in New York City, 2007–2011 (*Source*: Calculated from Table 3-2, p. 25, in Lobo and Salvo, *The Newest New Yorkers* [Lobo AP, Salvo JJ. The Newest New Yorkers: Characteristics of the City's Foreign-born Population (2013 edition). New York City Department of City Planning, New York: New York City; 2013]).

from Central America, while neighborhoods in Brooklyn have become home for a diverse mix of Chinese, Caribbean, Mexican, and Central American immigrants. Fewer of the new immigrants are settling in the Bronx or Staten Island (Lobo and Salvo, 2013).

Spotlight on Washington Heights and Its Dominican Immigrants

Washington Heights has been the community where most Dominican immigrants have settled, and it has the largest concentration of Dominicans outside of the Dominican Republic. Indeed, the neighborhood is known as "Little Dominican Republic." As shown in Figure 4.2, while Washington Heights has the largest concentration of Dominicans in the entire city, Dominicans are located in other parts of Northern Manhattan, particularly Inwood and Hamilton Heights, adjacent to Washington Heights. In Washington Heights, 60% of all immigrants are from the Dominican Republic, and in Northern Manhattan as a whole (from 125th Street and northward), they constitute 48% of all immigrants. In both Washington Heights and Northern Manhattan as a whole, the next largest origins for immigrants are Mexico, Ecuador, and other Latin or Central American nations. Only 14% of

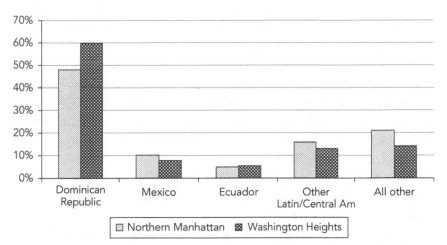

FIGURE 4.2 Foreign-born population 2011 by country of origin, Northern Manhattan and Washington Heights (*Source*: Calculated from Table 3-2a, Lobo and Salvo, 2013. Washington Heights is located at the upper north end of Manhattan, north of 155th Street, bordered by Harlem to the east and the Hudson River on the west. Northern Manhattan is all of Upper Manhattan minus Morningside Heights with its large university-related population of foreign students.)

immigrants to Washington Heights are from Asia, Africa, or Europe, while they are 21% of immigrants to Northern Manhattan as a whole.

Given that Washington Heights has a population which is half Dominican and other Latino immigrants, Dominican and Latino cultures are dominant in the neighborhood. Spanish is the lingua franca of the streets. Because of the high density of immigrants in Washington Heights, virtually any CHW program in this neighborhood will end up working with Dominican immigrants. Washington Heights is therefore an unusually appropriate neighborhood for exploring how CHWs can promote the health of immigrants.

The Heights, as it is known, includes the subneighborhoods of Washington Heights and Inwood, the latter located at the far northern tip of the island. Washington Heights has an economy dominated by retail trade, with supermarkets and grocery stores accounting for about 25% of all retail establishments. Most of the businesses in the Heights are small, with fewer than five employees, with the major exceptions of Columbia University Medical Center and New York Presbyterian Hospital, which have over 2,000 employees. Those who do not work in the neighborhood commute by subway or bus to jobs elsewhere in Manhattan or the nearby Bronx. The neighborhood is dominated by walkup apartment buildings, and 90% of the households are renters (DiNapoli and Bleiwas, 2008).

According to the US Census estimates, the Washington Heights population in 2012 was 263,281 (see Table 4.1). With a population that is two-thirds Hispanic, the neighborhood has one of the highest concentrations of Hispanics, almost three times the city average density of 28.6%. The immigrant character of the neighborhood is reflected by its population composition with half (46.6%) of all Washington Heights residents being foreign-born, compared to only 36.9% for New York City. Among immigrants, 83.1% are Hispanic, while significantly fewer are Black or African American, another difference from the racial/ethnic makeup of citywide immigrants, who are 32% Hispanic and 22% Black.

The US-born and foreign-born of Washington Heights differ according to several key characteristics that can affect their health and their ability to protect and sustain their health.

Compared to other foreign-born, Washington Heights has far fewer children. Most of the young children of immigrants were born here. This means that the immigrant parents will be protecting the health of US-born children, who will have access to insurance and other benefits that may not be available to their parents. At the other end of the age continuum, many more of the immigrants are seniors, aged 45–64 years or 65 years and over, both of

Table 4.1 Washington Heights-Inwood Population Characteristics, 2012

Characteristic	Total	US-born	Foreign-born
Total population	263,281	140,661	122,620
Under 5 years	5.5%	10.1%	0.3%
5–17 years	13.7%	22.0%	4.4%
18–44 years	44.8%	46.3%	43.2%
45–64 years	13.5%	8.4%	19.2%
65+ years	10.9%	6.3%	15.9%
Race/ethnicity			
Black	17.7%	21.9%	12.4%
Hispanic	67.4%	54.0%	83.1%
White, non-Hispanic	16.4%	24.7%	7.2%
Marital status (population >15 years)			
Never married	48.4%	66.2%	33.2%
Married or in union	28.8%	19.1%	37.2%
Divorced, separated, or widowed	22.7%	14.6%	29.6%
Educational attainment (population 25+ years)			
Less than high school	30.7%	13.1%	42.8%
High school graduate	19.0%	16.4%	20.8%
College or beyond	30.0%	47.7%	18.0%
Language spoken at home (population 5+ years)			
English only	29.2%	49.8%	7.8%
Other language than English	70.8%	50.2%	92.2%
Speak English less than very well	38.2%	8.4%	68.4%
Households with no one >14 years speaking English very well	24.0%	4.0%	39.3%
Economic status			
% unemployed (population >16 years in the labor force)	9.3%	10.6%	8.3%
Median household income	$39,475	$51,996	$32,921
Income at or below 200% poverty level	51.7%	47.0%	56.9%
Poverty rate for families (100% poverty level)			
All families with children under 18 years	31.7%	19.3%	36.9%
Female householder with children under 18 years	44.6%	31.5%	49.8%

Source: Compiled from American Community Survey, 2008–2012, zip codes 10031, 10032, 10033, 10034, 10040.

which have twice as many in this age group than among the US-born. These are the age groups of greatest importance when considering chronic disease risk, suggesting the need for programs to promote healthy lifestyles among immigrant seniors.

Compared to other foreign-born, Washington Heights immigrants are much less likely to be single and never married, while they are about two times more likely than US-born to be married, divorced, separated, or widowed. The high proportion of married couples suggests the need for family-oriented programs that will involve both spouses.

According to several indicators, even compared to other foreign-born, Washington Heights immigrants are at a significant disadvantage in terms of human capital and economic resources. Among adults aged 25 years and above, 42.8% have not completed high school, compared to 13.1% among US-born residents of the Heights, also well above the 28.6% among foreign-born citywide. Only 18% of the immigrants in Washington Heights have a college or postgraduate degree, two times lower than the 47.7% among US-born. The majority of the foreign-born in Washington Heights speak a language other than English at home (usually Spanish), and in 39.3% of households there is no one over age 14 who speaks English at least very well. Among the US-born, half speak another language at home, but hardly any are linguistically isolated. Here, too, it will be critical for any health program to be bilingual and to use materials that do not require a high level of education in English or Spanish. A positive approach for programs would be to integrate health and workforce development, so that immigrants can improve their health and their ability to compete in the labor market at the same time.

Related to their low level of education and language ability, Washington Heights immigrants are concentrated in low-wage occupations and their median household income is $32,921, far below the median of $51,996 for the US-born in Washington Heights, which is almost exactly the same as the citywide median household income of $51,865. Over one third of immigrant families and half of female-headed families with children under age 18 years have incomes below the poverty line. The immigrant families of Washington Heights are clearly the working poor, and programs must be designed that do not jeopardize their efforts to earn money and support their families. Activities need to be planned so they do not compete with work or school schedules. If they can be integrated into other income-maintenance or welfare-to-work programs, this will enhance the program attractiveness, at the same time that it supports the efforts of the community's immigrants to improve their lives.

Health Concerns of Washington Heights

Maintaining good health is likely to be a great challenge for many in this community, given their economic disadvantage and their vulnerability related to their linguistic isolation and constrained access to health insurance. As shown in Table 4.2, these constraints are borne out by the facts.

The health situation of Washington Heights residents is closer to that of all foreign-born in New York City, with some important differences. Washington Heights/Inwood adults are much more likely to rate their health as fair or poor, 32% versus 24% for foreign-born and 17% for US-born. The proportion that rates their health as fair or poor is closest to that for all Hispanic immigrants to the city, among whom 36% report themselves to be in fair or poor health. Washington Heights is also a community of fairly settled immigrants, and health status also declines with more years lived in New York City (New York City Department of Health and Mental Hygiene, 2006).

As expected given their economic disadvantage, residents of Washington Heights are much less likely than US-born city residents to have a personal doctor or medical home (32% versus 20%), and more have no insurance now or at some point in the past year (33% versus 9% among the US-born). While more Washington Heights adults are uninsured than among all immigrants to the city, they are only slightly more likely to go to the emergency department when they need health care, compared to all New York City US-born (9% versus 7%), but quite a bit less likely to rely on the emergency department for care than immigrants citywide (15%). Although the expansion of health insurance through the Affordable Care Act could reduce the proportion uninsured or having no personal doctor, a recent report from the New York Immigration Coalition finds that eligible immigrants are not signing up for insurance (Vimo and Weiner, 2013). Thus, access to care remains a significant issue for Washington Heights immigrants.

While they have higher rates of diabetes than both citywide populations, they are less likely to have high cholesterol and only slightly more likely to have high blood pressure than either group. Obesity rates in Washington Heights are 21%, identical to the rate for US-born New York City residents, but above the rate of 16% for all city foreign-born. Almost two thirds of the adult residents in the Heights do not exercise the recommended daily amount of 30 minutes at least three times a week, compared to 58% of the New York City residents. There is a need for diabetes prevention and self-management programs, but they need to be tailored to the particular patterns of cardiovascular risk found among this population, which in some respects is closer

Table 4.2   Health Status of Washington Heights/Inwood 2006 Compared to New York City, Total and Foreign-Born

Adult Health Indicators	Washington Heights/Inwood	New York City Foreign-born	New York City US-born
Health status			
Overall health rated as fair or poor	**32%**	24%	17%
Has been diagnosed with chronic condition			
High blood pressure	**27%**	25%	26%
High cholesterol	27%	32%	33%
Diabetes	**11%**	8%	9%
Asthma	5%	NA	5%*
Psychological distress	**10%**	7%	5%
Mental illness hospitalizations (per 1,000)	**13.2**	NA	8.1*
Health screening, risk factors, and prevention			
Has no personal doctor or medical home	**32%**	31%	20%
Has no health insurance now or in past year (adult <65 years)	**33%**	22%	9%
Go to the ED when sick or need medical advice	**9%**	15%	7%
Obese (BMI ≥30)	21%	16%	21%
Exercise 30 minutes daily for <3 days/week	**64%**	NA	58%*
Binge drinking in past month	14%	12%	16%
Birth rate among teens 15–19 years (per 1,000)	**106**	45	32
Child health indicators			
Childhood immunization coverage (4:3:1:3 at 12–24 months)	**63%**	NA	78%*
Asthma hospitalizations (per 1,000 children < 5years)	**10.3**	NA	7.2*
Asthma hospitalizations (per 1,000 children 5–17 years)	**4.3**	NA	2.7*

Note: Every bolded cell in the column for Washington Heights/Inwood indicates that their health status for that measure is inferior to the other groups.

Source: New York City DOHMH, "The Health of Immigrants in New York City, 2006." The data in these reports were collected using random telephone dialing to representatively sample adults in communities throughout the city, using an adaptation of the CDC Behavioral Risk Factor Survey. Asthma hospitalizations calculated from 2006 SPARCS data, NYSDOH. Immunization data are for 2002. North Manhattan rates are based on community provider surveys and New York City rates are from the National Immunization Survey 2002.

to the African American population than Hispanic or Mexican immigrants (Getaneh, Michelen, and Findley, 2006).

The residents of Washington Heights have higher rates of depression and mental illness than are found among the rest of the city's residents, US-born and immigrant. Because coverage of behavioral or mental health care is limited, relative to coverage for other health issues, obtaining adequate care is difficult even for those with health insurance. Combined with the absence of strong links to a medical home, this community's mental suffering is going untreated until it reaches a critical point, requiring hospitalization.

In the early 2000s, child health indicators for Washington Heights also lagged behind those for New York City. The childhood vaccination rates were one-third below the citywide average (63% versus 78%) (Findley et al., 2006a). Asthma hospitalizations for children were also way above the citywide average, and in 2006, the community's children continued to have higher than average rates of asthma hospitalizations (Findley, Rosenthal, et al., 2011).

Community Perspectives About Their Health Problems

In 1998, we began to work in the Washington Heights community to develop community-based approaches addressing their health problems. At that time the problem of access to health insurance was even worse than now, as this predated the expansion of the New York State Child Health Insurance Program (CHIP). In addition, the primary health care networks established by the two main hospitals serving the community, New York-Presbyterian Hospital and Harlem Hospital, lacked continuity of care and were not community friendly. There were virtually no prevention programs in the community, although they were much needed to confront the asthma and diabetes epidemics already affecting the community. Finally, many were concerned about dental and mental health care, both considered hard to cover, because many insurance plans gave little or no coverage for these services (Formicola, Perez, and McIntosh, 2012).

With support from the Kellogg Foundation's Community Voices program, we established the Northern Manhattan Community Voices collaboration, which included the lead partners of Columbia University's College of Dental and Oral Surgery, College of Physicians and Surgeons, and Mailman School of Public Health, New York-Presbyterian Hospital and its Ambulatory Care Network and Associates in Internal Medicine Group, Harlem Hospital Dental Service and Renaissance Health Care Network,

Community Premier Plus (managed care organization serving Northern Manhattan), Alianza Dominicana, Harlem Congregations for Community Improvement, and two dozen more community organizations and city agencies. The collaborative was deeply committed to the concept of community voice, to ensure that what we did truly reflected community views and would be implemented in full partnership with community organizations. We wanted to break away from the old style of university programs implemented by the medical center "for" the community, fully designed by the researcher with no input or say about the program from the community (Formicola and Hernandez-Cordero, 2012).

The Northern Manhattan Community Voices Collaborative established a Health Promotion and Disease Prevention Working Group to speak with the community residents and hear from them what they wanted in order to address their health concerns. In the words of the working group co-chair, Walid Michelen,

> We took nothing for granted. What were the main problems in our neighborhood? We could spout off a number of the usual diseases . . . But how did we know that this was really the case? We may think that our communities were interested in tackling these issues, but was that really the case?

The initial director of the Northern Manhattan Community Voices collaborative, Sandra Harris, underscored the importance of viewing the collaborative as an umbrella.

> Voices is an add-on, an umbrella organization. Voices provides an organization-wide vision, helping organizations to promote and advocate for some of the goals that we share in common. We do not want to be known only by the name "Voices," but rather by changes we bring about through the collaborative, the health insurance increases and changes in behavior and access coming through our partner organizations.

As part of the year-long exploration process, we collected 482 individual surveys, conducted numerous focus groups, dialogued with 13 community leaders, and completed numerous community health needs assessments. Surveys were taken of 48 community providers, and together with the New York City DOH Turning Point initiative, a community-wide dialogue was convened at which 225 community residents participated. Finally, we convened a community forum to review the findings from the exploration in order to select priority program areas.

The priorities identified through this process were asthma, heart disease and hypertension, vision or eye problems, nutrition and weight problems, domestic violence prevention, mental health and depression, and dental problems. In addition, everyone was very concerned about the need for health insurance, both among the uninsured who are eligible for insurance coverage and for those who do not qualify for any coverage.

The Washington Heights/Inwood community health survey conducted in 2006 shows that the health problems concerning the population had changed little between 2000 and 2006. Lack of insurance and access to care remained major issues, and the health problem areas identified continue to center around the chronic disease prevention and management, as well as of childhood asthma. Depression and mental health continue to be major burdens for the community. Thus, as the coalition initiatives evolved throughout the decade, we knew that they were still addressing priority health problems.

More important than identifying the health problem areas needing focused and coordinated attention, however, was the way that this priority-setting process involved the community and engaged residents in the process of developing the programs to address these problems. Reflecting on this process, Sandra Harris commented:

> It was wonderful to see the community's willingness to talk about the issues and direct us in the right direction about what they are looking for. They told us what they really needed. They went beyond the "stigma" issue to the real issues of living conditions, jobs, not just their mental status. We are whole people, and you have to consider the whole picture. Mental health is how I feel on a day-to-day basis, but my housing doesn't change. We should ask if we have always touched bases and looked at the comprehensive picture. The health promotion survey at Alianza starts with what services they need and then goes to the health and insurance questions. That is why people go there. At Northern Manhattan Housing Improvement Corporation, people are waiting at 7 in the morning because they are getting evicted. What we need is to work from there to include the health care and insurance program. We have to meet the community where it is at. Not just on health. Working with the community where they are at now.

Through this process we were able to understand the realities of people's lives and how little the facts about health care access told the whole story. It was not just having no personal doctor; it was also the feedback that the interactions with the system were so dehumanizing. Two immigrants participating in the focus groups said:

> Doctors were unfriendly, did not smile or speak to them, and cut their visits short. This made it difficult to trust the quality of care we received. Going to the doctor became the last option, to be avoided as much as possible.
>
> The doctors do not explain things or ask about decisions needing to be made. Since the doctors thought they [patients] didn't know very much, they ignored them. We don't feel that doctors understand our situation, the long waits and other problems we face as immigrants in the system. We are overstressed and frustrated.

Most telling about the health system was the following comment about how immigrants learned about the system itself:

> We learn about the health system by word of mouth, from our caseworkers, from posters at the grocery store or bus stop, or from street outreach workers. Word of mouth is especially important to us Dominicans. We like to share information and talk to each other, even with those we do not know personally.

Considering the combinations of the cultural and language barriers, the rushed and impersonal visits with doctors, and the sense that they were paying for every minute, is it any wonder that the many immigrants of Washington Heights lack a medical home?

Consistent with the goals of involving the community partners in establishing programs throughout the community to address the priority health problem areas, the Community Voices collaborative recognized that this required a new and different kind of approach. If the people's urgent needs were to be addressed, it meant that new bridges needed to be forged between the people, the organizations they trusted, and the health care system that they did not trust. We needed to integrate health initiatives into the social services, housing advocacy, immigrant rights, and educational programs offered at organizations and schools that people trusted. We could not work episodically; programs needed to be a part of the ongoing activities of the organization. This needed to be holistic, involving the whole organization—its leaders, its staff, its members—in the programs, so that the entire organization was committed to making the programs work. As a Community Voices Steering Committee member said:

> The behavior changes we envisioned take a long time. Health fairs are only one-time; we need continuous programs. We can't wait for people to come to the doctor, which is too sporadic and too late. Even when they are insured, people don't really use Medicaid, and they are afraid to come to the doctor except when the problem is serious or urgent, as they don't want to use up their annual quota of visits. We need to find more ways to go where the people are. The challenge is to get health education out of the doctor's office and into the organizations. The community's entire attitude to health care needs to be changed. Health care is not just a visit to the doctor; it is knowing how to shop, how to cook, what foods to eat. Why don't we agitate against fast food? McDonalds may be cheaper, but it is not better. Mental health is another big issue which the community needs to be involved in. The community needs to do it; all together we have to work on this.

Another Steering Committee member reminded us of the overriding priority of families to work together against poverty and to support each other to have a better life.

> To stand in great poverty in the shadow of great wealth is a burden of knowing inequities. Yet people have a great deal of hope. Parents have a deep longing for better, for more for the next generation. I cannot think of a guardian or parent who did not say I want more for my children than I have for myself. They weave their own nets, nets of compassion and concern. They do not have their own safety nets. With no safety nets we need to support each other and help one another. There is an excitement in seeing the weave of the web that is there.

From many different perspectives, it made sense for Community Voices to gravitate toward CHWs to weave together contributions to and from the community, engage residents in programs addressing health and social/economic needs, support immigrants learning about chronic disease prevention, and families new to the US health care system in navigating medical homes. Serving as a bridge between the community, its organizations, and the health care system, CHWs could ensure that people have someone they can talk with who they can trust to help them.

To make it easier for people to learn about health issues without sacrificing time needed for their other responsibilities, we decided to embed CHWs into the fabric of the community's social, educational, and economic services. The leaders at 11 partner organizations agreed with this approach, but they then needed to build their capacity to launch programs with CHWs. Half (55%) wanted to do this by expanding capabilities of their current staff, and another 27% by hiring new CHWs or peer educators, with the remainder not sure how to do it.

Thus, we adopted a strategy of integrating CHW activities into the work of our partner organizations, either by adding CHW responsibilities to existing staff or by bringing CHWs on board as new members of the organization's team. In this way, we would be able to reach the many thousands who did not have health insurance or did not use the health care system. Rather than waiting for them to turn up in need of urgent care, CHWs positioned within our partner organizations could reach out to everyone and engage them on health promotion issues, regardless of their connection to the community's health care system.

Northern Manhattan Community Health Coalitions

The first step in developing the coalition strategy was to hear in greater depth from the parents and community leaders about how they wanted to proceed. We organized coalition meetings that included representatives of over 14 organizations, and it became clear that the coalition wanted more than a single-purpose program. The Northern Manhattan Community Voices initiatives wanted a process that would enable them to develop, implement, and sustain the supports they envisioned. We began by developing a series of guiding principles, which were held in common by all Voices initiatives:

- By the community, for the community
- Put people first
- Integration of health promotion into ongoing social service/educational programs

- Community-based CHWs working directly with parents
- Evidence-based health promotion strategies adapted for the community
- Bridges to and from the health care providers
- Celebrate achievements

This next section of the chapter describes how we applied these principles, using coalition meeting records, activity reports, and the coalition's annual feedback and review processes, which elicited qualitative feedback from 254 parents and 102 CHWs over the decade of coalition activity.

By the Community, for the Community

The lead partner for our coalition activities was Alianza Dominicana, Incorporated. Alianaza's leaders, Moises Perez and Miriam Mejia, long had been inspired by Paolo Freire's "Pedagogy of the Oppressed", which stresses the importance of "going to the people" and building change from the ground up, with people articulating their most pressing needs and then transforming themselves and their community to address these needs (Freire, 1970). We had a strong commitment to making the program by the people and for the people, as articulated by Moises Perez:

> We need to get people involved in whatever language, so they feel part of it. We need to start from there. That's the important role of community organization: There's a great excitement in becoming part of wider society, of the greater spark. The community is cells coming together and working together, overlapping circles of strength.
>
> We are at the street level, open on the street, accessible all the time, helping people better manage their health and think about health. We want the community to be more integrated, working together around critical health issues, involving people with a wide range of skills and abilities and together seeing clear fruits of their efforts.
>
> We want a strong sense of ownership by the community. Community residents need to be in the steering committee. They need to have a real role in the community around this project.

Across three Northern Manhattan community health initiatives, Community Health Insurance Promotion (CHIP), Start Right (SR), and Asthma Basics for Children (ABC), we established a coalition structure whereby the community organizational partners were literally at the table, making decisions both large and small. CHIP included 4 community partners, SR included 23 organizations, and ABC included 31 organizations. The organizational members included multipurpose community organizations, immigrant rights organizations, New York City's CHW professional association, group and family day care providers, Head Start centers, elementary schools, faith-based organizations, local community health centers, and Columbia University's Mailman School of Public Health. We established a common mission for each coalition, developed the strategy and work plan together, and made budgetary decisions to allocate funds to each partner to support their work. Although the university and community health providers were partners, neither was a lead partner. The program coordinators for each coalition were based at the university partner, and they facilitated the organization of coalition-wide activities, such as trainings, monthly meetings, or community-wide events. All decision making was consensual, for large and small matters. The coalition agreed on the overall targets for numbers of people to reach and enroll in the programs, and held each member organization accountable for meeting its annual target.

Monthly coalition meetings were held at community organizations, with each partner taking a turn at hosting and leading the meetings. These meetings were attended by organizational leaders as well as any staff or volunteers who were involved in the project, including the CHWs they hired to work with them. A key function of these meetings was for the CHW to share strategies he or she used to work successfully with parents. Coalition members recognized and often gave prizes to the CHWs with the best ideas or who had the most success in the past month with outreach or follow-up. In Start Right, for example, we had a competition periodically for the most follow-up or reminder calls to parents whose children were due for vaccinations. This monthly sharing of lessons learned was vital not only in helping each organization meet its targets but also in enabling everyone to appreciate the outcomes of their collective efforts. Semi-annually, the coalitions reviewed their progress in achieving the overall health outcomes and celebrated their achievements.

Both Start Right and ABC had a Parent Advisory Board (PAB), which was led by one of the community partners, Northern Manhattan Improvement Corporation. The PAB met every other month and included two parents nominated from each of the organizational partners, who served on the board for a year. The CHW played a major role in recruiting parents for the PAB who could contribute based on their experience. The

PAB advised the coalition on a wide range of questions, including input to the design of appropriate health education materials to be used by the CHW with the coalition, strategies to engage health care providers, review of the logic models and grant application goals, recommendations for evaluation questions and methods, troubleshooting to help member organizations improve their outreach and engagement of parents, and semiannual feedback from a wider group of parents on how well the coalition was doing.

Putting People First

We heard from parents and organizational leaders loud and clear about their concerns for the health of their children, and we adopted the guiding principle of "Putting People First." We recognized that the challenge of working with the immigrant community was to connect to the deep desire among immigrant families for a better future for their children. Thus, the PAB turned the ABC mission of reducing asthma morbidity into "transforming parents' love and concern into effective care for their children." We saw the coalitions' activities as aiming to put parents in charge of their children's health. In the words of a member of the ABC PAB: "Only as parents become empowered can children benefit."

Empowerment for change is a participatory process, and if the coalitions were to be successful at empowering parents, we needed to do everything we could to make it easy for parents to get involved, participate, and, through this participation, take charge of their children's health. As four parents said:

It is not that we don't care. We do. We are busy. Please make it easy for us to participate in the program. Not too long or during the day when we work.

We want to do the right thing for our children, but we do not know where to go to find out what is needed.

I see other new mothers just sitting there and taking the appointment [for shots], and not realizing that it's important for their child to go once a month to get their shot and why. They don't know why they're taking them to the doctor, how many shots they're getting, stuff like that.

They don't want Medicaid. They don't feel they are eligible. They are working hard and they don't want Medicaid. They think Medicaid is welfare. They are worried about their legal status.

To make it easier for people to become involved and for the coalition to be maximally responsive to their concerns, each coalition incorporated into its strategies the following elements:

- Work with parents through the community organizations or programs that are already addressing their basic needs, such as faith-based organizations, day care programs, or schools.
- Reach parents through CHWs, who are best positioned to meet, engage, and support the parents on their own terms and within their own "comfort" zone.
- Provide options and choices for parents, so they can tailor their participation to their own needs and situations.
- Help parents get more out of their interactions with the health care system, and especially from doctors' visits.
- Help people organize information in ways that they can use it when they need it.
- Provide social support and positive feedback to participants, and enable them to talk to other participants so they can support each other.
- Provide educational materials and learning opportunities in ways that people can benefit from.

Integration With Community Social Service Programs

Along with the strategy of putting people's needs first, the coalitions endeavored to integrate health promotion efforts into existing community education and social service programs. Rather than adding yet another separate set of activities to the already complicated daily routines of busy families, we wanted to make it easy for parents by enabling them to participate in the program through their involvement in ongoing programs at community organizations, faith-based organizations, day care centers, or schools. This strategy was seen as critical to the objective of reaching many families with only limited external resources. It enormously facilitated outreach to the community, enabling word about the program to spread through the different existing organizational networks rather than being dependent on a single source, such as a hospital or a school. Families with children in need of the coalition programs were already coming to the social service programs, and information about the coalition activities could be easily incorporated into routine meetings and other interactions between the organization and parents. As a result, recruitment for the programs was able to reach deeply into the community. In the immunization coalition, for example, the integration facilitated a diverse recruitment from WIC sites (26%) and child care providers (20%), facilitated insurance enrollment programs (20%), parenting programs (19%), housing services (9%), and clinics (6%).

Rather than hiring and training a completely separate—and likely costly—team to promote specific health behavior changes, we opted to add health promotion activities to the existing programs of community organizations. We developed implementation guidelines to help each organization identify the best pathway and people for accomplishing the coalition goals. They were given flexibility to choose how to use the coalition tools and supports in order to accomplish the following basic activities:

- Identify potential participants, using simple screeners integrated into routine enrollment and review processes.
- Invite parents of eligible children to participate in group educational activities
- Support the parents in addressing barriers to change through one-on-one interactions with the CHW.
- Facilitate communication between the parent and his or her child's medical provider, including both health literacy activities and simple communication tools.
- Engage all children in educational activities, videos, and games to learn about their condition.
- Make their organization "health aware," for example, asthma friendly by reducing indoor environmental exposures.

The implementation guide was broken down into four or five different implementation strategies, one for each general type of partner organization: parenting programs, early childhood educational programs, schools, faith-based organizations, housing or tenant organizations, or community organizations (e.g., immigrant rights). Starting with the basic implementation strategy for their organizational type, each organization undertook a mapping process that helped them identify the best people and activities for accomplishing their share of the coalition's objectives. Because each organization had a finite budget, this strategy also was critical to facilitating an economical use of available resources. For example, instead of developing a separate screener for immunization status or asthma, a few simple questions were added to the organization's existing intake process. Staff members working with parents or children in diverse programs were trained to include the additional coalition activities in their routine work with families. Through this process the organizations took ownership of the coalition's agenda.

Consistent with the flexible approach of the implementation guide, the training also included team building, so that all the actors within the organization knew how their activities related to each other's work and to the larger objectives of the organization. In the asthma coalition, the day care provider/teacher handbook was a core resource that helped the teachers know where they fit into the entire program. While some thought they would be overwhelmed by additional training, the teachers wanted to know and be a part of the organizational change.

> The handbook concept, having everything in one place, meshes well with our desire as teachers to educate and share knowledge. It empowers us to speak about asthma one on one with parents. Questions about asthma management don't arise just at training; a handbook can be there to help whenever questions come up. I keep the handbook on my desk. It is my asthma bible.

Each organization developed its own work plan for how to work with its target population. Some organizations developed an additional group of CHWs who only worked on the specific goals of the coalition, but most integrated the activities of the coalition into a spectrum of staff and volunteers. The integration across diverse staff and programs created a wider net within the organization, enhancing the identification and enrollment of people from across the organization's many programs. Several organizations asked that all their staff, including office staff, be trained on the importance of childhood immunizations, and several of the schools and Head Start centers likewise asked that all staff be trained about asthma and how to respond if they observed asthma symptoms among children in their care. As one organizational leader said, "We have changed our organizational culture. Now everyone is attuned to immunization and we are all quick to identify and support parents to get their children immunized, regardless of their initial reason for coming to the organization." Immunization promotion, insurance enrollment, and then asthma control became embedded into the organization as part of their routine work, key to the sustainability of the coalition goals.

Community Health Workers to Promote
Health Behavior Change

It was clear to all the coalition partners that CHWs would be the prime agents of change. Although the community encompasses one of New York City's foremost hospitals, New York-Presbyterian Hospital, the issues we were addressing were better addressed in the community than in the hospital. Families are accustomed to go to the hospital for emergency care, being immigrant and Hispanic, but they seldom go there for anything less urgent, which meant that we needed another venue and other spokespersons to give the envisioned prevention and health promotion messages and support. Consistent with the vision of Alianza Dominicana, one of the lead partners in Northern Manhattan Community Voices, we felt that CHWs were key to this community-based strategy. Alianza had already built up a cadre of CHWs in their programs working with pregnant women, substance abuse, and violence prevention, so we logically turned to the CHWs as we began to develop strategies of health promotion for other topics.

Experience at Northern Manhattan Improvement Corporation and Alianza Dominicana had shown that ordinary people who became CHWs in Washington Heights were ideally situated to work within the community. Because their lives were already intricately interwoven into the community, sharing day care, markets, laundromats, schools, churches, and—being Dominican—favorite bakeries, CHWs who are immigrants themselves were ideally situated to build trust and confidence among their neighbors.

> I guess because I'm raised in the neighborhood—I wasn't born here, but I've been in Washington Heights all my life, I moved out and I've come back. . . . I guess I can identify with the problems that a lot of the families are having in the neighborhood. And being that I'm Hispanic also, and Dominican, that helps me out. Speaking Spanish definitely helps; it's a big part of making them feel comfortable.
>
> As Dominicans, we try to help each other, so whatever information has been useful for you, you try to give it to that person. So everybody that I know around, I try to give them information that's useful for them.

The CHW strategy was also consistent with our priority to integrate the coalition activities into the ongoing programs of each partner organization. Rather than imposing a new cadre of CHWs on top of existing staff, we worked with each organization to identify how they would grow or empower their existing volunteers and staff to be trained to become CHWs, often within the context of other organizational responsibilities. To give the organization flexibility in how it implemented the program, we developed a set of flexible CHW roles, allowing for variations in the amount of time a CHW would contribute to the work. As shown in Figure 4.3, the preferred strategy was to add CHW roles to those of existing full-time staff, followed by the more usual configurations of individuals recruited specifically to be CHWs.

- Full-time staff with CHW responsibilities added (n = 1,909): This group of CHWs was staff engaged for other program work to which the CHW duties were added. These staff had the advantage of already having a working, trusting relation with the parents, as well as regular times when they knew they would be interacting with them. This meant that they could make these interactions dual purpose, for the main program and for the health-specific activities, saving time for both the staff and the parents. These staff members were trained to lead meetings with parents and to incorporate other screening, educational, and adherence support work into their regular jobs. Generally, they worked in partnership with the part-time or volunteer CHWs, as they did not do direct outreach.
- Part-time paid CHWs (n = 474): The next level up was composed of part-time CHWs who received a small stipend. Because many of the CHWs were busy parents with young children, part-time work suited their personal schedules. These part-time CHWs did outreach with other families at their organizations, as well as helping to organize and support

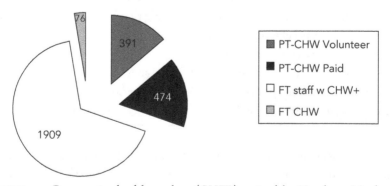

FIGURE 4.3 Community health workers (CHWs) trained by Northern Manhattan community voices coalitions, 2000–2010.

small meetings with parents. Many spent hours making phone calls to families to remind them about immunizations or to come to the next parent education session at the organization.

- Volunteers (n = 391): Some organizations had a large pool of potential volunteers, so we developed a set of activities for volunteer CHWs who worked only 5–8 hours per week. As peers already known to people they were contacting, the volunteer CHW roles concentrated on outreach to parents and reassuring them of the value of participating in the program.
- Full-time CHWs (n = 76): Finally, there was the smallest group, CHWs hired full-time to work only on the coalition's agenda. These CHWs had the most extensive set of responsibilities, including health coaching, role-playing to share experience, and informal counseling and support.

Across all the coalitions, the majority were either full-time staff with CHW responsibilities incorporated into their work, part-time paid CHWs, or a mix of volunteers and full-time CHWs. If organizations spread CHW responsibilities across multiple categories of volunteers and staff, we helped them make sure that activities did not get overlooked.

Regardless of their level of engagement with the program (volunteer to full-time), all CHWs were trained using a similar comprehensive process that built their core competencies, along with their ability to support families to make the recommended changes in their health behaviors. Training was conducted by the program managers and faculty members of the coalition, and every training session was organized to teach both content and how to engage and teach the parents about each specific content area, building in a train-the-trainers approach for all participating CHWs. All CHWs learned how to use appropriate communication techniques to engage parents, including those who were fearful and those who were perpetually rushing off. The trainings were participatory, and the CHWs were coached on how to apply this participatory method when working with parents. Interactive role plays were used to ensure that CHWs could use appropriate verbal and nonverbal communication techniques that would encourage parents to participate, ask questions, and learn. The CHW trainings were incremental, with each successive training building on the experience gained between each training session and enabling the CHWs to progressively expand their activities from outreach to coaching. Based on the responses of the 84 CHWs included in the New York City CHW surveys 2007–2010, by the end of the sequence of training 85% or more of the CHWs in these coalitions had developed competencies in the following core competencies:

- Development of a trusting relation
- Listening
- Multicultural communication
- Facilitating goal establishment
- Health education or coaching
- Informal counseling
- Case management
- Advocacy
- Outreach
- Event/workshop organization
- Information exchange techniques

Fifty percent or more had developed competencies in an additional eight core competencies. Here is a sampling of feedback that CHWs provided on the core competency skills training they received, across all three coalitions.

> Basically it taught us how to communicate with people, not to talk down to them. They may come for Medicaid, but we learned effective listening, how to listen for key words to identify what other needs they might have. So, I listen to them, give them as many referrals as possible, and follow up frequently.
>
> We are trained to deal with a lot more than the case managers do, which is mainly clinical and telephone follow up unless deemed medically necessarily. We communicate with parents and address their problems. We don't just make referrals; we work with the families. At our community organizations, we feel that we are not by ourselves and have resources. We feel that we are not alone and we can reach out and find resources for our patients.

The coalitions spent months developing health education approaches tailored for the immigrant community with whom they would be working, and these approaches were built into the CHW training modules of each coalition. Each coalition provided topic-specific training in a series of 4–6 modules that covered basics about the health problem, specific skills needed to educate parents about what they need to address this problem, use of audiovisual or other tools to assist in educating the parents, specific steps needed to link the parents to their primary care provider, and monitoring and follow-up activities specific to each coalition. The coalitions selected culturally and age-appropriate audiovisual materials that were approved by our

Parent Advisory Board and well liked by the community. The CHWs were trained how to integrate the use of these audiovisual tools with their personal communication, such as stopping the video and having a Q&A about the last segment seen. In this way, the CHWs were able to use high-quality health education materials without having to become health education experts themselves. For example, the Start Right immunization coalition developed a bilingual brochure to educate parents about the dangers of not vaccinating their children by incorporating the CDC images of people with preventable diseases and pairing them with messages about the diseases and how shots prevent them, drawn from other CDC vaccination education materials. The ABC coalition developed bilingual parent handbooks, "How to control your child's asthma," incorporating New York City and national asthma education program messages, but tailored in shortened messages with pictures so that the handbook could be used by people with limited reading abilities.

We also developed active learning tools that would help parents visualize and understand through their own movements, such as the "asthma fist" to explain how the lungs contract and spasm during an asthma exacerbation, just as one squeezes the hand shut when making a tight fist. The handbook contained several games that could be played with preschoolers to help them learn about asthma and asthma triggers, and all the teachers at the day care centers and schools were trained in using these games. We trained the CHW to offer a variety of activities that could be tailored to the needs and time constraints of the organization and parents, such as showing the asthma video with a Q&A that could be viewed at the time they were picking up their children, reminder cards, parent workshops, club cards that incentivized accomplishing the recommended asthma control activities, and simplified pictorial asthma action plans making use of stickers portraying the child's prescribed medications. In this way, the CHW learned how to be effective at communicating with parents, regardless of the parent's literacy level. Those who made home visits were given additional training in how to initiate and conduct a home visit in a supportive, nonthreatening manner while still remaining safe themselves.

This is what the day care providers had to say about the training in using multiple educational methods for parents and children:

> Before, I didn't have enough information to know how to care for children with asthma. Now I can help our parents to understand better and how to deal with asthma if they have a child with it.

I didn't know anything. I learned a lot. I learned to avoid the triggers, to have the children get tested to see if they are allergic to certain triggers, and to see which symptoms they have. I learned how to work with the child who has asthma and recommend to parents that they go to the doctor and get medications.

They gave me a video from *Sesame Street* [A is for Asthma] and I put on the video. It tells about what the environment has to do with asthma. The children love it.

We stressed throughout our meetings and trainings that the highest priority for the CHWs was to prioritize the needs and concerns of the immigrant families. As immigrants themselves, many with experiences of negative interactions with the health system, the CHWs were coached on how to support the immigrant families in a nonthreatening way, to be flexible to the families' concerns. The whole tenor of the interaction between the CHW and participant was expected to be one of support for addressing the participant's concerns and helping the participant become empowered to address them. CHWs were expected to be coaches, facilitating problem solving by the families. Here is what three CHWs had to say about being responsive:

It is difficult to go into people's homes, inside their comfort zone, and tell them how to make changes, even if it's for the good of their children, because that implies that they don't know how to take care of their child or know what's best for their kids. The main challenge for me is the sensitivity to people. I can't always do what is put down on paper as that can be a little unrealistic.

I go into the community making home visits to help people understand and manage asthma, but there are times when you have to do more. As a CHW, I want to be somebody who can change something . . . to give people the tools to be self-sufficient.

Sometimes they have personal problems. They have economic problems. There are people that don't have their residency documents, and one feels useless, incapable. These problems touch me because I'm human. And you want to help them in every way possible, but we can only help them in one way. At least I can give them strength. And there are places that can help them, so I recommend them to go there. We can give them letters to go to the church and get food.

Thus, rather than insisting that there was only one fixed set of educational sessions or activities that the parents needed to do, the CHWs and organizations were encouraged to be flexible, giving parents choices for when and how they engaged with them. For example, while home visits were an important part of helping families with asthma learn what to do about asthma triggers in their own home, the asthma coalition CHWs were trained *not* to insist on a home visit if the family did not want one. Educational videos were shown at the time when parents were picking children up from day care or school, so they could be caught "on the fly" if the parent had missed an evening group educational session. Parent mentors were available regularly at the entrance to the schools or Head Start centers if parents had questions.

The location of the CHWs in the community, at day care centers, schools, churches, or much-accessed community organizations, made it easier for the CHWs to set up appointments to see people or, conversely, for people to find them. This location also enabled people to take advantage of other supports and connections possible through the organization. At Alianza Dominicana, for example, a Center for Health Promotion and Education was established on the ground floor of its headquarters, and within that space the organization built an indoor replica of a traditional Dominican healer's home and invited visitors to go in. The organization's walls proudly displayed masks and other crafts produced by the community's youth. Upstairs, a large open area was turned into an art gallery where the community's artists were invited to display their work. Thus, those coming to see the CHW at the community organization could visibly feel the CHW's roots in a shared immigrant background and culture. Recognizing the value of being able to refer families to the coalitions' own programs, we prepared a list of social service programs available across all coalition members.

Evidence-Based Health Promotion

We developed culturally and community-appropriate educational and communication tools based on accepted principles of health education and health behavior change (Green and Kreuter, 1999).

- *Proper diagnosis of the problem:* As described earlier, we listened to community members, teachers, day care providers, organizational leaders, health care providers, and CHWs to understand the priority problems and then delved deeper with additional formative research to identify across the different interconnected layers of community and health care system the specific barriers to health behavior change among the immigrant community.

- *Hierarchical:* We trained the CHWs to start by eliciting people's concerns, and not to assume that the health problem they were concerned about was a valid concern of the individual. Their support was organized in a logical way to help the individual progress from awareness to action by way of understanding, motivation, and preparation for making changes.

- *Cumulative learning:* Materials and communication strategies were developed to build on prior learning. Parents were introduced to the concept of asthma medications only after they had learned something about asthma as a disease, and children learned about triggers only after they understood that the coughs that some of them had were asthma episodes that could have been triggered by animal dander. The schedule of immunizations was introduced only after parents understood and wanted their children to be vaccinated.

- *Participation:* Whether working with immigrant parents or their medical providers, the educational process was designed to be participatory, using interactive teaching techniques appropriate for adult learners. CHWs were trained to engage participants, to get them talking, to validate their wisdom and to use role-play methods to help describe the desired behavior changes. When we showed a video, the CHW ended the viewing with a group discussion about the film and what aspects of the film corresponded to his or her own situation. Similarly, the training for physicians emphasized culturally appropriate communications and stressed the need for the providers to engage and stimulate participation by the patients.

- *Situational specificity:* There was no lack of education and communication tools for promoting immunizations or asthma self-management, but our coalition found that they could not be used "off the shelf" in this community. We translated, rewrote to simplify and reduce the reading level required, added more pictures, including ones of families from the community, and integrated the messages into activities and "products" that were familiar to the families. The Parent Advisory Board and the CHWs reviewed all materials and tried them out to make sure they could be used effectively with the immigrant families. For example, we developed a "club card" that parents could use to check off their accomplishments in gaining control of their child's asthma. When they had completed at least three of the recommended steps, they went to the CHW with whom they were working and could claim a gift prize, such as an age-appropriate book for their child to read.

- *Multiple methods:* Achieving the desired changes to immunization coverage or asthma control required many changes, not just by the parents but also by the system. After diagnosing the problem, we mapped out change strategies pertinent for each aspect of the problem. These diverse changes were implemented in a coordinated fashion, so that as the CHW was working with individuals, the system would be "ready" to respond appropriately when the participant began to change. For example, asking parents to bring an asthma action plan for their child to the child's day care provider did no good if the physicians did not make out a plan for the child with the parent. Providers needed this training before the parents were asked to make this change. Whenever possible, we introduced innovative communication and support methods that would shift the supportive system to a new level and one which made it easier to support behavior change, such as a system-wide immunization registry accessed through the Internet in each provider's office, electronic versions of the asthma action plan in the electronic medical record, or an interactive query-and-answer tool that physicians could access in their consultation rooms to answer questions about asthma or immunizations. Similarly, as noted earlier, the asthma coalition developed bilingual handbooks for the day care teachers and staff to use in explaining asthma symptoms and control to parents.

- *Individuation:* Across all the communication and coaching strategies, we emphasized the need to tailor the material to the individual. Instead of simply giving parents a copy of the immunization schedule, the CHWs were trained to look at the child's immunization card and to advise the parents on what shots their child still needed and when. With the parents, they completed a simple sheet, "When the Next Shots Are Due," clearly indicating when the parent should take her child for immunizations. Then, the CHW would call to remind and encourage the parent a week before the immunizations were due. This individuation approach was wildly successful, as parents soon learned all the immunizations schedules and assumed responsibility for their completion. This community empowerment was most rewarding to the coalition and all parties involved. Similarly, we developed a simple pictorial asthma action plan to help explain the doctor's plan for parents, clarifying the time of day when their child should take daily medicine—and a picture of which one—and when to take "relief" medication, again with a picture of which medication to use. Because the coalition also wanted children themselves to learn about asthma control, we developed games and activities like an annual poster competition to make it fun for children to learn about asthma and asthma triggers.

• *Feedback:* Overlaying all the CHW activities was the emphasis on giving feedback or social support for the immigrant parents. The CHWs were trained to provide positive reinforcement and support to families whenever they made steps toward change. All progress, large or small, was celebrated. Each organization had a process by which they convened parent meetings or support sessions where the parents would have the opportunity to ask questions and to hear how others had solved problems. The feedback principle was also applied to supervision and support for the CHWs. Monthly coalition meetings provided an opportunity to share lessons learned. When progress was lagging, we brainstormed on additional things we could do to expedite change. This feedback component helped draw out extraordinary individual and group capacity, nurturing the development of permanent leaders and community organizers among the program participants and partner organizations.

Bridges to and From the Medical Providers

Recognizing the importance of appropriate health care for the attainment of the coalition goals, health care providers were partners in the coalitions. Unlike many health-related coalitions, however, the medical partners were not the lead partners, and from the start we emphasized the need to build bridges to and from the health care system. CHWs were the primary bridges promoting a healthy interaction between the community members and the medical providers. For this bridge to be effective, it needed strong supports on both sides of the bridge.

On the health care provider side, we worked with the health care provider networks to make their services more immigrant friendly: providing extended hours and weekends, and bilingual staff, including physicians, bilingual educational materials, welcoming office environment, and timely services. We worked with the city and state agencies to connect the health care providers with training and supports for state-of-the-art care practices: a Web-based immunization registry and electronic medical records with prompts to remind physicians about key questions to start a dialogue about immunizations or asthma symptoms and severity. In addition to training sessions organized through the hospitals, we worked with the primary care providers throughout the community to disseminate the latest evidence-based clinical guidelines, along with training in how to apply the guidelines. In partnership with the medical providers, we developed culturally appropriate educational materials for the health care providers to use in their practices, and we distributed the coalitions' favorite videos to show on the televisions in the waiting rooms.

On the community side of the bridge, we implemented a number of activities supporting a stronger connection between community residents and the health care system. In partnership with the facilitated enrollment initiative of Community Voices, our coalition members referred the uninsured to enrollers to help them sign up for health insurance. The CHWs learned about the different neighborhood providers available per plan and helped families to choose a medical home. To encourage people to make visits to the community physicians, we invited the physicians to coalition meetings so that the CHWs and community residents could meet them and see the human and immigrant-friendly face of community providers. We organized periodic "Ask the Doctor" sessions at local partner organizations, so that CHWs and community residents could ask questions in a setting in which they were most comfortable. We promoted primary care visits, not just for the mandatory health examinations for day care or school admission but for well-child visits and asthma "tune-ups." We showed videos to promote health literacy, demonstrating how to go to the doctor and ask questions.

Overlaying all these efforts was our emphasis on promoting improved and supportive communications with medical providers. We met with the medical providers and developed supportive tools that would facilitate better communication between the immigrants and medical providers. In the case of the immunization coalition, this included providing immunization information materials in a low-literacy, bilingual format, along with educational sessions led by the CHW to answer questions and prepare the parents for the visits to their child's health care provider. For the asthma coalition, we provided the Physician Asthma Care Education (PACE) training. PACE is the NIH-recommended training program that trains physicians in assessing asthma severity, models effective strategies for establishing a trusting relation with the patient, and then shows how to jointly develop an asthma action plan with the patient's family, so that the family can understand how to use prescribed medications appropriately to manage asthma flare-ups. With the assistance of our immigrant pulmonologist and pediatrician partners, we added culturally appropriate role plays that specifically focused on how the health care provider would speak with immigrants, including use of body language that would be welcoming and nonthreatening. We did role plays with the physicians to help them learn culturally appropriate ways to convey their recommendations to parents.

Over the project lifetime, we trained 276 out of 306 pediatric primary care providers in our community, and we tracked changes in their asthma management practices before and after the training. After training, providers were more likely to use the recommended asthma management tools and skills. The greatest increases were in regular classification of asthma severity, from only 35% prior to the training to 83% after the training. Appropriate use of controller medications for children with persistent asthma increased from 61% to 95%. Physicians also reported an increase in their discussion of environmental triggers with patients, from 5% prior to the training to 41% after completion.

At the same time, we developed a series of communication tools to help prepare the immigrant parents for their visits with the doctors. We asked the physicians what questions they thought parents could ask if they wanted to learn more about their child's illness, and we then integrated these questions into the parent educational sessions, giving the parents a "Club Card" with questions they could ask, so that the harried and flustered parents would have reminders of their questions when they had their 7 minutes with the doctor. Parents overwhelmingly liked the card, and it has now been reproduced in many formats, including a short version printed onto a key holder.

Implemented separately in the health system or community, these changes were unlikely to have brought immigrants flocking to the health care system. What was needed was a change in norms about using the health care system, and this is where the CHWs were instrumental. Perhaps the most important aspect of bridging the gap was the work of the CHWs to dispel myths, answer questions, and share positive experiences, essentially building trust in the community for the health care provider. In group sessions the CHWs encouraged people to talk about how they overcame their fears and received much-needed help from one of the community providers. More than anything else, the CHWs provided the gentle push and support that helped families overcome their hesitation and distrust and actually go to the doctor. Complementing this normative shift, the CHWs coached people on what to expect in a doctor's visit and gave them tools such as the asthma questions to take with them. In educational sessions, the CHWs translated the medical terminology and recommendations into language that the immigrants could understand. The following exemplifies how CHWs saw their role in facilitating these communications:

> Sometimes the doctor–patient interaction prevents patients from getting care, because the thing about the hospital here is that the people don't have enough time to spend with their patients. They have to see somebody in 5 minutes and fill the papers and that's it, you see? And most of the patients, they don't feel comfortable asking questions because they know the time, like they say, time is money here in the United States, and they don't feel like they have enough time to ask questions and be familiar with the doctor and ask the doctor questions. The big issue is time. To do more home visits would reach more immigrants than currently, because sometimes, the people have issues and they don't know how to express the issue, but when you come to them, they open to you, they express the necessities that they have, and you can help them in a lot of ways. We explain about asthma and the medications in ways they understand. Now, when moms go to the doctor they know what is going on and understand what he tells them. So, they come back and thank us for helping them understand.

As a result, parents became empowered to ask the questions that unlock the information flow and communications between the parents and the physician.

> I used the Club Card. It was useful because it helped me remember things that I should be doing and also because I could remember to ask the doctor questions. I didn't know what asthma was or what questions to ask. The club card was my guide. I asked my doctor how often I can give my child quick-relief medication, and he initialed every question I asked him. He took the fact that I wanted the card initialed seriously. The card helped me keep track of successes.
>
> They teach us how to ask the doctor. I think that is important, because we do not know what the consequences of the medications are for children, and now we can ask the doctor about it.
>
> I learned how to inquire about the vaccinations my baby should get. I asked my doctor more. I had been anxious that the vaccine has viruses. I felt that giving the virus would be harmful. The doctor told me that it was okay because you get immune to it.

Celebrate Achievements

Our last guiding principle was "Make it fun!" We wanted both parents and children to have fun while learning about immunizations or asthma.

- For immunizations, we adopted a two-step communication strategy: first to show pictures of what the various diseases looked like to give them a sense of reality, and then to explain the child's vaccination card and demystify the vaccination process. When the child received the next round of vaccinations, the CHW would call the parent to congratulate her, and when her child became up to date she received a certificate honoring her achievement.

- In the asthma coalition, we designed a whole set of educational games appropriate for 2–8 year olds, adaptations of well-known games like Match-Me or Twister, but with the content being asthma triggers. Both teachers and parents were taught how to use them and instructions were included in the ABC handbook series. We selected fun videos for preschoolers and elementary school age children to view to learn about asthma, and actually used the one for school children as a staple in our work with parents. The "street-wise" minority youngsters in the film *Roxy to the Rescue* were easy to understand and easy for both parents and children to identify with. Showing the film never failed to elicit comments and subsequent questions from the audience.

- For many years, the asthma coalition sponsored a poster competition to coincide with World Asthma Day. In the months before the competition award ceremony, the CHWs went to the day care centers and schools and worked with the teachers to show the asthma videos, engage the children in the asthma games, and then provide them with the materials for making posters to enter into the competition. Hundreds of children submitted entries each year, totaling 3,335 submissions from 2004 to 2008. The award ceremony was attended by up to 300 people gathered together to admire the posters and celebrate with the winners. The award-winning posters were displayed at the participating schools and selected New York City art galleries. Finally, the asthma coalition sponsored an asthma walk in which over 200 families participated as part of a community "Climb the Heights" event to promote walking in the neighborhood.

In both coalitions, we held annual Christmas parties for the families, which became festive opportunities for everyone to have fun together, and in the asthma coalition we added "graduation" ceremonies in the spring to celebrate the accomplishments of children who had gained control of their asthma after a year of care coordination by the CHWs.

Along with these family-oriented activities, the coalitions also sponsored public feedback events where community members were invited to celebrate the accomplishments of the coalition. Sometimes these were integrated into the graduation or poster competition events, but otherwise they were complimentary events, where parents could see how their own efforts to support their children's health contributed to advancing the health of the neighborhood. In addition, the coalitions shared progress toward attaining their goals with their Parent Advisory Board, who shared it in turn with their parent organizations.

Community Health Workers Working to Improve Health in Northern Manhattan: How It All Worked

Between 2000 and 2010, the three coalitions within the Northern Manhattan Community Voices Coalition recruited and trained a total of 2,850 CHWs. During the decade in which these coalitions were functional, the CHWs reached out to 167,457 individuals, screened 82,226 for their health care needs, found 50,726 to be eligible for services from the coalition's CHWs, and enrolled 44,677, who then received support from the specific program's CHWs.

While only 440 of the CHWs worked in the CHIP-facilitated insurance enrollment program based at Alianza Dominicana, they were supported by a huge cadre of student summer volunteers and women participating in the Welfare to Employment Program (WEP), who distributed flyers widely in the community. With this help they did outreach via flyers, health fairs, and visits to community service sites, such as WIC, reaching over 100,000 persons (see Fig. 4.4). About half of these came in to be screened for eligibility, for which 33,623 were eligible to apply for themselves or their children. With the assistance of the CHWs at Alianza and its partner organizations, 30,000 adults and children were enrolled in Medicaid and the state's Child Health Plus program.

Start Right had double the number of CHWs ($n = 998$) and with some additional assistance from the summer youth employment program participants, they reached 31,156 parents of children under age 2. About one third of these followed up with the CHWs to have their child's vaccination cards read

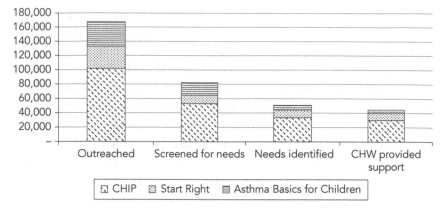

FIGURE 4.4 Outreach, screening, and enrollment into the Northern Manhattan Community Voices coalition programs, 2000–2010.

and vaccination needs determined, and 90% of the children were determined to be not yet fully vaccinated. Virtually all of these parents (n = 10,251 or 97%) enrolled in the program and received support from the CHWs in bringing their child's immunizations up to date (see Fig. 4.4).

Asthma Basics for Children had the most CHWs (n = 1,412). They were able to do outreach to 34,438 parents through an extensive array of presentations at schools, day care centers, health fairs, WIC and income maintenance sites, parenting programs, community clinics, churches, and other community organizations. Of those who heard about the program, half completed the coalition's short screener to determine if their child had diagnosed asthma or its symptoms, which were found in 6,563 of the children screened. Two thirds (67%) of their parents enrolled in the program and received support from the CHWs.

The key step in engaging the community was the personal contact between the CHW and the parent during which the child's eligibility for services was assessed. In all three coalitions, about half of all persons who heard about the coalition program actually followed through with the CHW to find out if they and their children could participate and receive support from the CHW. When they sat down with the CHW face to face to find out if their needs could be served by the coalition, almost two thirds (62%) were found to be in need, and of these almost all (88%) enrolled in the program to receive support from the CHW. In explaining this remarkably high participation rate, the CHWs observed that the personalized screening process was itself educational for the parents. As they were reviewing the family's situation, the CHWs were able to explain more about the problem and what the coalition could do to help address their family's health needs. By the time the family's needs were identified, they were already convinced by the CHWs that they could do something about them if they participated in the program. Indeed, CHWs often observed that as they were doing the screening, the parents had their "Ah, ha!" moments when they understood what the problem was and that they could do something about it.

By the time I'm halfway through the application, I know a lot about the children's health, other problems, the situation in the household, 70% of the time. Sometimes, I see something is wrong. I tell them we have counselors here and say, "Here's my card. Call me and I'll call back." Once I make them laugh or smile, it helps a little bit.

I have used the asthma web site (asthmabasics.columbia.edu) with one child who was diagnosed. After alerting the mom, we used the web site to educate her about asthma. She had a big aha moment!

Our families face so many other challenges that asthma is at the bottom of their list. They are facing eviction, losing Medicaid, domestic violence, and other issues. The fact that we, the family asthma workers, are trying to get the parents to look at and address asthma for their kids is a challenge.

It was the fact that there were a lot of things in their lives at the moment, and they were not interested in taking care of their asthma at that moment. It was the last thing on their list. So I was trying to help them with asthma, and it was a lot of work to get them to the point of taking asthma seriously. People were at different places in terms of stages of change with regard to asthma. The social issues were the biggest concerns for people, and this was difficult.

The CHWs were encouraged to be in touch with families often, and every organization developed its own strategies to make it easy for the CHWs to reach out to the families. In addition to home visits, they made phone calls to check in with their clients, greeted them when they dropped their children off at day care or school, helped them make doctor's appointments, and invited them to small group workshops. Generally, there was a shift from home visits to phone calls over time, as shown for families whose children received asthma care coordination in Figure 4.5.

The CHWs were highly motivated to follow up with the families, and they appreciated being given options in how they could reach them. The average number of personal or phone interactions per enrolled family was 5.1 for

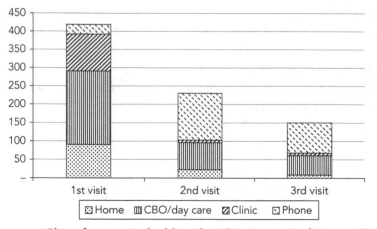

FIGURE 4.5 Place of community health worker–client interaction ($n = 437$ asthmatic children enrolled in care coordination).

Start Right and 5.3 for the ABC coalition, while those receiving care coordination in the ABC coalition received an additional 2.9 phone calls or visits. Here is how two CHWs in the Start Right program describe their continual efforts to reach families:

> We work here as a family, so it's a good structure. We do everything we can to encourage them to complete the application. We call them, mail them, do home visits if they live in the neighborhood, have parties, meetings. We do everything. I don't know what else we could do. If we see them in the street, we even remind them.
>
> Families only bring children in when they're sick. So they don't understand the whole well-being of the child completely, that it's okay for them to come in when they're not sick and have them checked out. They do not understand that; they think we just want to take their money. But it's not that. And they think that they don't deserve better and that they can't better their lives. So it goes a little deeper than just the appointment for immunizations. So, I use the reminder about their appointment and the information that I give them as a hook, to boost their morale a little bit. I need persistence. I call the parents often, and usually I go to their home. We're in their home, and usually they feel a little bit more comfortable, so they'll open up a little bit more. It's so important in their home, where you can build more of a personal relationship with them.

In both the Start Right and ABC coalitions, we conducted annual feedback surveys with a sample of parents, generally through the school or day care as part of end-of-year events or at one of the coalition celebrations. Across all the years, we obtained feedback from 836 parents participating in the immunization coalition and from 1,133 parents participating in the asthma coalition. The parents were very positive about the program and actually thought it should be expanded to reach more working mothers like themselves. Here are some examples of what they had to say about what they learned from the CHWs:

> I did not know about children's vaccines. I like the information we got about the diseases you get when the children don't get vaccinated. Because of the program, I learned to read my child's immunization card. I realized my child needed more shots. The program helped me to make and keep appointments for the rest of my child's shots. I think the program did all that they could. The rest is up to me.
>
> My son had problems breathing all the time in Mexico, and the doctor said it was flu. But when he got sick here, the doctor said it was asthma. She explained it to me, but I didn't understand. When I heard about the ABC program, I came to a workshop. They explained everything. Now my son takes the medicine and isn't sick all the time anymore.
>
> They explained asthma to me with more detail than the doctor tells me. The training helped me to follow the treatment plan the doctor gave me, because before I was doing the treatment the wrong way.
>
> When my child first had an asthma attack, it was scary and I did not know what to do. But now I am able to know when the attacks are coming. Oh what a difference!

The CHWs worked through a combination of individual and group interactions, and our data analyses and feedback from parents showed that those who participated in the group activities got more out of the program. The following quote from a mother who participated in the Start Right coalition through her child's Head Start program illustrates how the CHW's individual attention helped the mother to get more out of her participation in group activities.

> First of all, they gave me an invitation for a meeting that they had at Ft. George [Head Start program]. And I went to that meeting to learn about the program. They told us that if our children were 1-year old they should

have their vaccinations already, that they need their vaccinations as part of a normal development. I learned that in this country, you have to have shots to get children into school. Then a different day I went to the office to ask them a question. I went to ask about a program that I saw on television about a child that got sick from a shot. She became abnormal, her brain seemed to be fine, but her body became deformed. So I was concerned and went to ask. At Ft. George Alexa [the CHW at Ft. George] gave me a pamphlet about shots and explained it to me. Alexa told me that she couldn't say that it was the shot, but neither could she say that it wasn't the shot. It could be that the child had the problem before she got the shot, and the mother just thought that it was because of the shot. That made me feel better about getting shots for my child. This is a good program, because parents have to be reminded every month. I know that anything I need they are there to help me out. I have gone twice to ask them questions. They always tell me that anything I need, they are at my service. They respond right away. Alexa always calls me before I go to the doctor and also afterwards. The only thing that I would say is that they should keep on working in this. Just as I didn't know, there are many mothers who don't know about the program and they need it. It's important to keep promoting and informing people about it so they can benefit as well.

In their personal outreach to parents, the CHWs stressed the importance of the group events when the parents would have the opportunity to see the educational videos, but also when they could talk with other parents to learn how others had resolved issues they all faced. In the ABC coalition, participants watched the "Roxy to the Rescue" video an average of 2.9 times, and they participated in 2.3 group workshops. Again, the effect of providing a space and time where parents could learn from each other and ask questions was an extraordinary change in their encounters with the health care system – one that created new norms and expectations for the participants. Here is feedback on the importance of the group sessions:

We let all parents know when we were going to have the asthma workshop, and the parents came out pretty good. It was good that all parents can come, because even if they don't have a child at day care with asthma they may have a sibling, parents, or grandparents with asthma. So it is very useful for everyone to be invited. Then, when they are asking questions, it means they are involved.

They invited us to a meeting with all of the mothers and they explained that we need to know what they are putting on the [immunization] card, because one often doesn't know. This makes one more careful and aware. So you are always checking. For me this is very good. I love the idea of the class they give us. They taught us how to read the cards and to see in which months the children need to get their shots.

They put me in touch with other women and we shared opinions. That helped me to get stronger and be more independent and got my mind positive before it became negative.

I would say that this is a place for moms where you can educate yourself about your children and meet other moms like you. They can benefit from the program when they work together.

In both the Start Right and ABC coalitions, the parents learned how to play an active role in keeping their children healthy, and it is clear from the feedback from parents that the CHWs played a lead role in helping them to learn what they could do. In the case of Start Right, the key elements they learned were how to read their child's vaccination card, to use the New York City vaccination schedule to determine if the child needed another shot, and then to make and keep appointments with the doctor to get the shot(s). Here is how one woman described how the CHWs helped her accomplish these steps.

I went to a meeting with other mothers to learn about shots for my baby. They explained about shots and showed us pictures of the diseases they could get if they did not have shots. And then they explained about going to the doctor. "They'll give her this shot and that shot ... make sure that when they give her the shots they mark it in your card." These are things that possibly one knows, but it is better to get all of the information. That way they are telling you, "Look, this is what is happening. This is what you need right now."

Then they [two CHWs from her daughter's Head Start program] came to my house once when the baby was 1 month old. This visit helped a lot. I have my daughter, but when she was born things were not like this. Things have changed. They explained everything, step by step. From that point on, they made sure I was up to date. I see them every day when I go to drop off my daughter, so they ask me when I see them how I am doing, if we are up to date. They ask me to bring in the card for them to see. Sometimes I forget, but when I bring the card in, they check it and make photocopies. They tell me, any doubt you have, let us know. I've already consulted with them twice. They check the card to be sure the child is up to date. They have it under control and are always checking in.

They gave me gifts, little things for the children. The gifts are nice, but they are not the most important thing. The most important thing is the attention they give me. They are so kind. They think more about what you need to do than you do yourself! More than what they have done I think they cannot do. The women are so pleasant and this is very important. It gives you trust. You open up because you trust them and then you feel free to ask whatever you want. One learns a lot. Isn't that what life is about? When they offer me things like this, I go because one learns.

Similarly, the parents participating in the ABC coalition were immensely appreciative of the support they received from the different CHWs, whether they were part-time volunteers, the parent asthma mentors, or full-time trained CHWs who provided more intense support and care coordination to help them bring their child's asthma under control. Here is what four parents said about how the program helped them:

My son's asthma is easily triggered regardless of what is done to prevent attacks. I had tried home remedies, but they didn't help. I took him to the Dominican Republic for some home treatments, but he came back worse. The program has given me insight into how to manage asthma and prevent it. Now that I am in the program I am more comfortable about medicines. I liked how the asthma worker [CHW] went through the information step by step and explained about the medications. There was so much to learn: triggers, meds, prevention. I made repairs and had an exterminator eliminate roaches. I learned that there are different types of medication, for an attack and for prevention (three pills). The program helped me to talk to the doctor. I feel more knowledgeable. I feel I know more about the medications and am on top of them. I no longer wait for my child to have an attack to give him the pump. I learned about prevention.

The asthma worker has changed my life. Before getting involved in the asthma program, I visited the emergency room at least 10 times a year. The family asthma worker cleared out some doubts I had. I had asked my physician, but felt more comfortable with the asthma worker. The asthma worker has also taught me about asthma medicines and has cleared up the doctor's instructions on how to administer the medicines. I was finally able to understand. My daughter has not had an asthma attack since she started the program, which is a year ago.

At the beginning I felt bad because I didn't know what to do, and now I feel good because I do. My son was 7 months old when he got asthma. It was very difficult and it was a very bad experience for me. I wasn't sure if he was going to live. I now give Singulair to him, and since I started using it he hasn't gotten asthma. I am a mother who now knows what to do ... I feel sure of what I do and how I treat him.

I learned to have confidence in myself when my daughter has asthma. I try to be calm and react better so I can manage my child's asthma and help her. The training helped me to spot her asthma signs and know what to do.

Those who had the additional benefit of care coordination from a CHW were more likely to lack confidence in managing their child's asthma at the start of the program, 47.9% versus 34.8% among those whose children had less severe asthma. After 1 year in the program those with intensive support for care coordination *and* those with less intense support through a combination of activities led by CHWs both had a 43% gain in confidence in managing their child's asthma. In the mixed support group, the changes in use of controller medications and the asthma action plan were the greatest, with controller medication use rising from 38.5% to 47.8% and having an asthma action plan from their doctor increasing from 36.7% to 46.6%.

The ABC coalition follow-up surveys specifically asked those who received individualized support from the family asthma worker ($n = 379$) how participation in the coalition helped them better manage their child's asthma. As shown in Figure 4.6, it is clear that the participants appreciated the blend of activities, with the group workshops being considered the most valuable.

The coalitions assessed the outcomes of their activities using indicators linked to the primary goal of the coalition, and across the board the coalitions were successful in helping parents improve the health of their children. As shown in Table 4.3, there were significant improvements in the community health indicators addressed by the coalition.

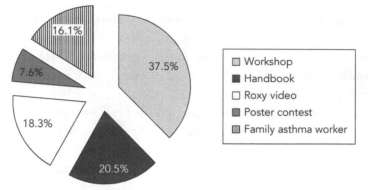

FIGURE 4.6 Which ABC activities most helped you?

- Insurance coverage rates for eligible children went up by 47% and for eligible adults by 122%.
- Childhood immunization rates rose from 63% to 97%, a 54% increase that exceeded the city and national averages, 76% and 80%, respectively. In fact, this intervention eliminated one of the most glaring disparities

Table 4.3 Community Health Indicators Targeted by Northern Manhattan Coalitions, Before and After Coalition Activities

Health Indicators	Status at Coalition Launch	Status at Coalition Termination	Percent Change
Insurance coverage rate (<17 year olds)	64.4%	94.7%	47%
Insurance coverage eligible adults (18–64 years and living in poverty and not recent immigrant)	33.1%	73.4%	122%
Childhood immunization coverage (4:3:1:3, 12–23 months)	63.0%	96.8%	54%
Asthma hospitalizations (per 1,000 children <5 years)	10.3	4.1	−60%
Asthma hospitalizations (per 1,000 children 5–17 years)	4.3	1.7	−60%
Asthma ED visits in past year (per 1,000 children <5 years)	47.6	34.9	−27%
Asthma ED visits in past year (per 1,000 children 5–17 years)	20.0	18.0	−10%

in the country. It is not often that we can reference the elimination of a health disparity. Between Healthy People 2000 and Healthy People 2010, even the federal government reduced their expectations from "eliminating" disparities to "reducing" them. Yet, here we have the extraordinary experience of eliminating a major disparity.

- Childhood asthma hospitalization rates declined by 60% and emergency department visits also declined. By the end of the coalition's activity in 2010, the rates were at or below the New York City 2010–2012 averages for childhood asthma-related emergency department visits, 35.5% for children <5 years and 20.4% for children 5–17 years, and the asthma hospitalization rates were below the city averages for both age groups, 7.8% and 2.9%, respectively.

In addition, ABC also assessed changes in asthma management among those parents who participated in the program. As shown in Figure 4.7, after only 1 year of participation, parents receiving support from ABC's CHWs experienced significant reductions in their children's uncontrolled asthma episodes. There was a 60.0% reduction in asthma-related emergency department visits and a 60.6% reduction in asthma-related hospitalizations for those in the mixed CHW group (*n* = 2,213), while in the group receiving care

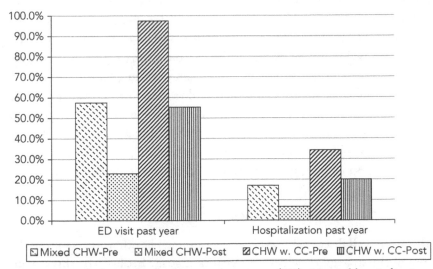

FIGURE 4.7 Asthma-related emergency department (ED) visits and hospitalizations at enrollment (Pre) and 1-year follow-up (Post) for participants in ABC by type of community health worker (CHW) support.

Table 4.4 Asthma Management by Level of Participation in Community
Health Worker–Led Workshops

	No Workshops	1 Workshop	2+ Workshops
Asthma management outcome	$n = 493$	$n = 205$	$n = 110$
Easier to talk to the doctor	37.4%	81.7%	86.0%
Reduced triggers in the home	82.9%	89.0%	90.6%
Got asthma action plan from doctor	13.9%	53.4%	67.2%
Took AAP to child's school	33.5%	49.8%	55.5%
Confident managing child's asthma	81.0%	92.4%	90.4%
Reduced emergency department visit frequency	57.3%	67.7%	58.7%
Reduced hospitalizations	80.8%	91.4%	90.9%

coordination from CHWs ($n = 217$) the comparable reductions in emergency department visits and hospitalizations were 43.2% and 41.7%, respectively.

Accompanying these changes in basic disease management indicators, there were significant increases in the proportion of parents who adopted the recommended asthma management practices. As recommended by the CHWs, 78.1% of the parents had spoken to their doctor about asthma, and 88% reported that it was easier to talk to the doctor after participating in the program. The proportion of children with moderate-to-severe asthma who were prescribed controller medications rose from 50.1% to 59.7%, and the proportion with an asthma action plan rose from 37.3% to 46.8%. Participating parents' confidence in managing their child's asthma rose from 64.0% to 80.2%. Almost all parents (93.6%) knew about environmental triggers to asthma, and 89% had taken steps to identify and remove triggers in their homes. Those who participated in the group workshops were more likely to make changes in managing their children's asthma, as shown in Table 4.4.

Conclusions and Reflections

Throughout all three coalition efforts, community health workers were at the core of the strategy to achieve the coalition goals. Because the three coalitions evolved out of shared visioning, we were able to learn from each other's successes and failures, and thereby strengthen the involvement of CHWs in promoting the community's health. Almost 3,000 CHWs were recruited, trained, and supported to work on behalf of the coalitions' agendas. They touched the lives of 167,457 individuals, and worked directly with 45,000 individuals, most of them immigrants or the children of immigrants. And they were immensely successful. The results shown in Tables 4.3 and 4.4 demonstrate the effectiveness of the CHWs in reaching, engaging, and nurturing the immigrant families to improve their children's health. In addition to the strong contributions to the health of the community's families, feedback from the participants showed that the CHWs were helping families become empowered in many ways, not just accomplishing one or two of the recommended behavioral changes. The families were overwhelmingly supportive of the CHWs and were deeply grateful for the support they gave to making changes and getting connected to the system. As many recounted, if it had not been for the CHWs, they would not have become insured, gotten their children immunized, or brought their children's asthma under control. More important, the parents speak with pride about their accomplishments. What they learned strengthens what they are able to give to their children.

What are the lessons that we have learned for how the CHWs have helped them cross that seemingly formidable bridge to improved health care?

- *Organizational base in the community*: Consistent with the vision of the Northern Manhattan Community Voices, all three coalitions were based in the community with up to 32 partner organizations. This gave the coalitions a wide base of operation, enhancing the potential to reach deeply into the community. The design and implementation of the CHW strategy was the result of collective thinking across the partners, not imposed by the health care system or academic partner. The partners owned the coalition activities completely. In all partner organizations, the organizational leader valued the CHWs and encouraged their staff to welcome the CHWs and their work. Without this support it would not have been possible to integrate the diverse CHW activities into the heart of the organization's daily function.
- *CHW options:* The coalition gave organizational partners options for how to incorporate CHWs into their activity flow. Most chose to add CHW roles to the work responsibilities of existing staff, for example, day care providers or family support workers in parenting programs, and they saw this as a "win-win," enhancing their staff capacity to support families without having to add another layer of workers. However, these staff-cum-CHWs were supported by a diverse network of CHWs, ranging from volunteer to full-time, and they all worked together as a team.

- *CHWs as immigrants:* The vast majority of the CHWs were immigrants themselves or else the children of immigrant parents. They used this experience to gain the trust of families and to demonstrate possibilities for change. When CHWs spoke of doing outreach in the community, they were talking about walking in their own neighborhoods, among people who came to know and respect them for their work. Community members knew where to find the CHWs and vice versa.
- *Fully trained CHWs:* Regardless of their level of effort, all CHWs received training in basic core competencies, not just the specific content area related to the health outcomes pursued by the coalition. Feedback from the CHWs and from the parents, as well as the outcomes, show that this core competency training was invaluable for the attainment of the coalition goals, both in recruitment but more important in following through and supporting families to make behavioral changes.
- *Health providers as partners:* In all three coalitions, the CHWs needed to know community health providers who would be able to respond appropriately to the immigrant families when they came for care. The coalitions provided training in communications and support for electronic records or other tools that would make it easier for the providers to welcome and relate to the CHWs. The coalition gave providers culturally appropriate flyers and videos that they could show to parents, and they invited community pediatricians to community forums and meetings so parents could ask them questions. At the same time, we received advice from the medical providers about how to best coach families on immunizations or asthma control, and these best practices were incorporated into our training and tools. But we also made it clear that the community groups were leading the coalition, not the health care providers. This made it possible for CHWs to "bridge the gap" on their own terms, linking the families to the providers in a gradual process that built trust in the providers.
- *Embedded in the community:* Many CHW programs are funded by short-term grants and do not have the time to become a part of the community. We worked hard to have multiple sources of funding over almost a decade, and this enabled the CHWs to become established members of the community. In addition, the organizations that added CHW roles to the work of existing staff had basically provided themselves with a stable and sustainable cadre of CHWs. Many of the CHWs in one of the coalitions worked in the others, and this also provided a stable sense of connection.

As will be discussed in the next chapter, the coalitions have continued to evolve, both to continue the same set of activities and to expand into new areas of need. In the next chapter we will include several of these in the discussion of alternative CHW organizational models.

While the coalitions were remarkably successful in achieving their goals of improved health care for the immigrant families of Washington Heights, there were several challenges that we were never fully able to overcome. The next generation of coalitions will undoubtedly need to address these challenges in order to more fully reach all the immigrants.

- *Monitoring and data sharing:* The coalitions had to develop creative strategies for tracking the activities of the CHWs and the impact of their work on health outcomes. Despite having IRB and HIPPAA approvals from participating parents for access to medical records, the hospital system made it very difficult for the CHWs to access or share information about the patients with whom they worked. We had to develop an independent data "warehouse" to keep track of immunization data when the hospital backed out of prior arrangements to allow the CHWs read-only access to the immunization registry via our collaborating pediatric partners. We had to ask the parents for copies of the child's asthma action plan, as it was not possible for the CHW to view these online, although subsequently arrangements were made for this through the emergency department. CHWs also had no way to directly inform pediatricians about patients they referred to them. The indirect methods we developed to track outcomes sufficed, but it would have been easier if the CHWs at least had read-only access to relevant portions of the medical record. We demonstrated that they were fully competent to read and evaluate immunization cards, and it is not unreasonable to anticipate being able to develop a template that a CHW could use to download critical information about patients they see.
- *CHW turnover:* There was a fairly high rate of turnover among the CHWs as they took new jobs or transitioned into different roles as their children progressed from day care to elementary school. This was particularly an issue for the volunteer and part-time CHWs. We therefore combined training and refresher courses on an annual basis, to ensure that all organizations had trained CHWs supporting the coalition's work. Related to this was the issue of salaried work for immigrant CHWs who do not have work permits or residency status. We did not want to put organizations at risk for violations, and therefore we had to be flexible about the involvement of volunteers.

- *Women dominated:* Perhaps because of the focus on health problems of early childhood, most of the CHWs (98%) and most of the participants were women. We had male CHWs in one of the programs, but they were not welcomed on home visits, so we shifted to all women for the home visiting roles. This gender imbalance may have affected the involvement of men, and if programs want more men to be involved, they will need a more gender-balanced cadre of CHWs.
- *Mental health issues:* Many of the parents we worked with suffered depression or other forms of mental illness. These were beyond the counseling ability of the CHWs, and in future programs it will be important to expand the role of the CHWs to support depressed persons and link them to the mental health care system.

5

Program Models for Community Health Workers Bridging the Gap

IN NORTHERN MANHATTAN, the feedback we received from CHWs and community residents suggested that it really made a difference where the CHW had her home base. Many CHWs preferred to be working at community organizations, where they felt most comfortable, but those who worked within larger organizations, such as the hospital, appreciated the advantages such a structure gave them, particularly in reaching people who most needed their help in managing a chronic illness such as asthma. Within the coalitions we identified distinctive configurations for the institutional base for CHWs: health facility, community organization, or local county or city government. This diversity of organizational "homes" for CHWs highlights the importance of thinking about organizational structure and the links between the CHWs and the organizations. This chapter focuses on the organizational structure for employing CHWs and how each organizational structure may lend itself to supporting CHWs in their work with immigrants. It will move beyond the Washington Heights community to include a wider variety of settings and programs in New York City and beyond, with a view to fleshing out the operational details that contribute to the success of each of the three basic models.

Organizational Options for Employing Community Health Workers

In the preceding chapters we have focused on what CHWs do to promote immigrant health, but where they are located within the organizational structure makes a difference to how and what they are able to do. There are three basic organizational models for hiring and supporting CHWs:

1. Employed by a health facility
2. Employed by community organization
3. Employed by government agency

Examples of each of the three basic models are given in Table 5.1. This table also shows hybrid models combining two of these models with shared hiring and supervision.

To provide a more in-depth perspective on how CHWs work with immigrants in each of these models, we conducted additional interviews with the leaders of selected programs: Bronx-Lebanon Family Medicine (Romelia Corvacho and Douglas Reich), NOCHOP (Letty Guzman) Asthma Basics for Children and WIN for Asthma (Sally Findley and Patricia Peretz), NYU-RICE (Nadia Islam and Jennifer Zanowiak), NYU-DREAM, CSAAH and ASPIRE programs (Nadia Islam and Lindsey Riley), Hennepin County DICE (Nathan Ellis), Salud para su Corazon (Hector Balcazar), and Poder es Salud (Noelle Wiggins). These interviews were supplemented with information from published articles about each program.

Employed by a Health Facility

In this model, the health facility recruits, hires, trains, and supervises the CHWs. They are employees of the health system, which puts them inside the medical care team. This means that they need a niche within the medical system hierarchy, and the usual possibilities are to be linked to the system via the social worker line of command or through nursing, but they may also be part of community medicine, a system-wide resource "on call" or seconded to clinical services, as in the WIN for Asthma program of New York Presbyterian Hospital. Examples of the health facility model are shown in column 3 of Table 5.1.

There are several advantages to this organizational structure:

• *Enhances CHW–medical provider communication:* With the CHW inside the health system, it is easier for the CHW to communicate with the medical team, including the doctor, and vice versa (Peretz et al., 2012). The CHW can set up a regular time to meet to exchange information about patients. In addition, there are more opportunities for the healthcare team

Table 5.1 Examples of Community Health Worker Programs by Institutional Base for Community Health Workers

Health Facility or Health Plan	Community Organization	Government Agency	Mixed Model (Facility + CBO)
Health Plus, NYC (Thimot, Martinez, and Matos, 2004)	Northern Manhattan Community Health Worker Outreach Project (Palmas 2014)	Erie County Cancer Screening Outreach (NACCHO, 2014)	Asthma Basics for Children, New York City (Findley et al., 2013)
Bronx-Lebanon Family Practice (Findley et al., 2014)	Start Right, New York City (Findley, 2006)	Hennepin County, MN DICE project (Ellis, 2014)	WIN for Asthma, NYPH and CBOs (Peretz et al., 2012)
Care Guides, Allina Hospital, Minneapolis, MN (Adair et al., 2012)	Salud para su Corazon, Texas (Balcazar et al., 2011)	Poder es Salud, Portland, Oregon (Farquhar et al., 2008, Wiggins 2009)	La Red de Asma Infantil-San Juan, PR (Lara et al., 2013)
LA VIDA, Hidalgo Medical Services (McCloskey, 2009)	Santa Clara Co. Vietnamese PAP screen outreach (Mock 2006)	Healthy Homes-Seattle-King County, WA (Kreiger et al., 2005, 2009)	Starr County border diabetes initiative (Brown et al., 2002)
Promotora diabetes program, El Paso (Lujan et al., 2007)	HELP-PD Diabetes Prevention Program (Katula et al., 2011)	NYC East Harlem Asthma Center of Excellence	Be Active Together, Seattle-King Co. (Marinescu et al., 2013)
Patient Advocates for Asthma, Philadelphia (Apter, 2013)	SDMP, San Francisco, CA (Lorig, Ritter, Villa, and Armas, 2009)	NYC Managing Asthma in Day Care (Sale-Shaw, 2013)	Cambodian "whole health model, Lowell, MA (Grigg-Saito et al., 2010)
Child Asthma Link, CHOP, Philadelphia, PA (Coughey et al., 2010)	ENLACE physical activity promotion, Texas &SC (Messias et al., 2013)		Hepatitis Outreach to Foreign-born, New York City (Perumalswami et al., 2013)
Familias Sanas PostPartum visits, Phoenix, AZ (Marsiglia et al., 2010)	Entre Amigos, Yuma County, AZ (Nuno et al., 2011)		NYU-RICE initiative w. Korean immigs. (Islam et al., 2013)
Cancer screening outreach, Florida farmworkers (Wells et al., 2012)			Community-based breast health navigators, CA (Nguyen et al., 2011)
La Clinica del Cariño, Oregon (Volkmann and Castanares, 2011)			

members to get to know each other and to build relationships of trust and understanding. With time and the trust it brings, the CHW may be able to make suggestions to the medical provider that will facilitate his or her interactions with immigrants, as happened at the Bronx-Lebanon Family Medicine (Findley et al., 2014).

- *Integration of the CHWs into the primary health care team:* Many primary care practices are moving toward developing a patient-centered medical home or the more expansive health home. Having a CHW member of the primary care team facilitates the communications and support necessary to make the team truly patient centered and patient responsive (Adair et al., 2012; Findley et al., 2014; Markova, Mateo, and Roth 2012; Volkmann and Castanares, 2011). The health system can support this integration through interprofessional training that enables all team members to better understand and support each other's roles (Fronek et al., 2009). A common model within the medical system is to have a nurse supervise the CHW and thereby anchor the CHW's care coordination within the health care team, as in the example of the adaptation of the Yes We Can model for asthma care coordination to meeting the needs of families living in housing projects in San Juan, Puerto Rico (Lara et al., 2013).

- *Direct lines of authority within the health care team:* When the CHWs are hired by the health system, they become members of the health care team. They occupy a niche within the team with clear lines of supervision from the medical, nursing, or social worker chains of command. This makes the CHW accountable to the structure, but it also means that these structures are obliged to supervise and support the CHWs. The health system's Human Resources office can provide a structure through which to recruit, train, and hire the CHW (Lara et al., 2013; Peretz et al., 2012). However nurse supervision of CHWs also runs the risk of diluting the CHW voice, a lesson learned from the Family Medicine program at Bronx-Lebanon Hospital.

- *CHW protocols and activities well defined:* When there is a team of CHWs working in the health care structure, they need a clearly defined division of labor, so that they can be integrated into the health care team. This clarifies the responsibilities of the CHWs and also alerts the other members of the team to what they can expect (Lara et al., 2013). Some of the protocols may be more limited, such as following up with patients seen in the emergency department, while others may be quite extensive, such as when the CHW is part of a patient-centered medical home or providing care coordination services (Adair et al., 2012; Coughey et al., 2010; Lob et al., 2011; Thyne and Fisher-Owens, 2011).

- *Comprehensive training:* When the hospital hires CHWs, it typically provides the CHWs with a comprehensive CHW training as part of their orientation. Comprehensive training includes core competencies related to the CHW scope of practice, tools and material tailored for CHW support for patients with particular diseases, topics, and employer-specific processes such as implementation of research protocols, forms, HIPAA and IRB considerations. In more successful CHW programs, the initial training may be for 70–110 hours, covering the core, disease-specific, and employer-specific skills (Findley et al., 2014; Ruiz et al., 2012). At New York University Medical Center, CHWs hired to work with diverse immigrant groups on different health issues were all provided with a comprehensive training program with all three types of training. At Bronx-Lebanon's Family Medicine Department, the training was given to a larger group of qualified candidates and their conduct during the training was one of the factors used to determine those who were actually hired.

- *Gives the CHWs status within the health system:* As an employee of the health system, the CHW can be trained and provided access to clinical areas or hospital information systems that outside CHWs might not have access to. For example, with access to the scheduling system, the CHW can facilitate coordination of visits and then follow up with the patient. Some health care systems also have given CHWs access to the electronic medical records so that they can directly share information about the patient with members of the health care team (Fagman et al., 2011; Findley, Rosenthal, et al., 2011; Rosenthal et al., 2006).

- *CHWs can serve as patient navigators:* CHWs are often hired by hospitals to help patients navigate the system, particularly cancer patients with multiple tests and doctors' visits. Working within the system, they can track when a patient is due for a visit so they can call and remind them, and then they can follow up after the visit. In the case of Denver Health, the CHWs supplemented these simple reminders and calls with discussions about barriers so that they could work with patients to overcome their barriers (Nguyen, Tran, Kagawa-Singer, and Foo, 2011; Perumalswami et al., 2013; Raich et al., 2012; Wells et al., 2012).

- *Funding is institutionalized:* If the hospital is hiring workers, there is a greater likelihood of stable funding, as in the case of the CHWs being hired for WIN for Health by the New York-Presbyterian Hospital, which is using its own funds to hire them. Within the health system, it is also possible for the hospital to reimburse CHWs using insurance capitation fees. This provides the system with a stable cadre of CHWs, which is easier for the hospital to manage, since it is time consuming and disruptive of care if CHWs are laid off every time there is a funding shortfall. In addition, when the hospital makes a commitment to cover the salary of the CHWs, they are much more invested in integrating their services consistently in the health system (Findley et al., 2014; Peretz et al., 2012).

• *Facilitates referrals to and from the CHWs:* As members of the health system, the CHWs have more complete information about social work services or other specialized services that their clients may need. They can work directly with the social work staff in making and following up on referrals. The social work staff rarely has time to follow up with patients, so this support increases the chance that the patients will make use of the referral. Further, the CHW can find out if the referral was helpful and, if not, work with the social work team to remedy the situation (Coughey et al., 2010; Lob et al., 2011).

• *Possibility of a career ladder:* With a large enough cadre of CHWs, the hospital can organize regular trainings that enhance the skills of the CHWs. Some CHWs can become senior CHWs, mentoring those newly trained, and the senior CHWs can become supervisors within the CHW team. In the Family Medicine Department at Bronx-Lebanon Hospital an experienced CHW managed the CHW program, reporting directly to the medical director (Findley et al., 2014). This last model was purposefully developed, because the medical director wanted direct access to what the CHWs were discovering and feared that placing a "clinical" person in management of the CHW program would dilute that information. If the CHWs are employed within a health care plan, it is also possible to organize a similar training and structured mentoring and supervision program.

These advantages come with some not insignificant disadvantages:

• *CHW no longer seen as belonging to the community:* CHW activities and roles may tend to become "medicalized," and they might be seen as unapproachable for the same reasons that people do not talk to nurses as they do to CHWs.

• *Distrust of the system:* CHWs located in the health system face being less accessible to community residents, especially immigrants who are deeply distrustful of the "system."

• *Inaccessible to uninsured:* People without insurance will not know about or access CHW services through the health system.

• *System barriers:* Guards at the doors and the need to show ID are a big "Keep Out" sign to immigrants.

- *Square peg in a round hole:* CHWs are not a known workforce within the health system, and human resources may not find it easy to create appropriate positions or recruitment policies. Position descriptions may emphasize education and training, biasing against CHWs who are community-wise though with low formal education. The hospital may see the CHW position as a place to "dump" low-skilled employees being laid off from other positions, as happened at Bronx-Lebanon Family Medicine.

Employed by a Community Organization

This is the most common model for CHWs working with immigrants. After receiving funding, the community organization specifies the CHW roles and activities to accomplish the program goals, and then recruits the CHWs from the community. CHWs may be full- or part-time. Some of the CHWs may be current staff of the organization who take on CHW functions. The community organization generally provides training for the CHWs, and they are supervised internally. The CHWs use the community organization as their operational base, frequently making referrals to programs offered by the organization. The CHWs in this model may or may not work closely with medical providers, but generally with less direct contact than for CHWs employed directly by the health care facility. Several of the diabetes prevention and control initiatives illustrate the model of CHWs being hired, trained, and supervised by community organizations, usually, but not always, several of them (see column 2 of Table 5.1).

There are many advantages to the model with CHWs employed by a community organization:

- *Easy access to and by community:* Being located at the community organization means that the CHW is located right within the community and therefore readily available to community members. This is particularly important for people with limited income who would not seek services if they incurr transport costs (Balcazar et al., 2009; Fernandez et al., 2009; Katula et al., 2013; Lorig, Ritter, Villa, and Armas, 2009; Peretz et al., 2012).
- *Credibility of the community organization:* The community organization where the CHWs work may be recognized as a trusted place where immigrants can go for help, as was seen repeatedly for immigrants consulting the CHWs at Alianza Dominicana in Washington Heights (Formicola et al., 2012). The process of building trust with the CHW is facilitated

by the presumption that a trustworthy organization has trustworthy staff (Farquhar et al., 2008; Shah et al., 2013).

- *Organizational network and resources:* CHWs are continually seeking programs and resource persons to help their clients, and those working at a community organization often benefit from a diverse array of programs and networks that can be tapped through the community organization (Formicola et al., 2012; Perez and Martinez, 2008).
- *Collegiality:* While the CHWs may be isolated as the "only" community people in the health system, at the community organization they are working with other community members. The team is all around them, and the CHWs can easily find collegial support and friendship among other staff, if not among other CHWs themselves.
- *Familiarity with CHWs:* Many community organizations have relied on CHWs for years, and they have built up experience working with CHWs. In this setting, supervisors understand and can better support the CHWs in their work (Formicola et al., 2012).
- *Flexibility:* Community organizations often have a less rigid structure, and this benefits the CHWs who need flexibility regarding scheduling visits with clients according to their availability. CHWs may also have more flexibility in how they support the clients with whom they work, which can help them to be more responsive to their client's needs (Findley et al., 2006a).

Despite all these advantages, there are several disadvantages that CHWs face from an operational base at a community organization.

- *Weak or absent link to medical providers:* CHWs based at community organizations may have difficulty forging links to medical providers. As a consequence, it may be difficult for the CHW to bridge between the community and the health system.
- *Work overload:* Community organizations often try to implement a program without a full complement of staff or resources. As a result, the CHWs can easily become overloaded, to the point that they cannot meet the organization's expectations. There may also be some blurring about responsibilities of the CHW, with the CHW possibly being expected to take on responsibilities beyond his or her scope (May and Contreras, 2007).
- *Insufficient human resources:* Organizations, especially small ones, may have a limited budget for training, and as a result the CHWs may be asked to begin working after a short training. The training may not include the core competency skills, such as communication, counseling, or coaching.

In addition, unless the organization has a large number of CHWs, training is likely to be done by available training resources, which may or may not meet the needs of the program. Lack of supportive supervision can be another issue for CHWs working at community organizations, if supervisors are unfamiliar with the work of CHWs and unable to support them in improving their skills.

- *Funding insecurity:* CHW positions at community organizations are usually grant funded, and if the funding disappears, so may the CHWs. Thus, the CHWs at such organizations experience a higher level of job insecurity and anxiety about the loss of funding (Peers for Progress, 2014).

Employed by Government Agencies

Many CHWs work directly for the city or county or a government agency in a program serving the needs of immigrants (inter alia). A variant of this model is for the CHWs to be employed by a partner agency, such as a hospital or multiservice community-based organization, while still being funded, trained, and supervised by the government agency. As with the CHWs employed by the health facility, the governmental agency uses a standardized process of advertising and recruiting for CHWs, and they may even have a career ladder for CHWs or public health advisors, as they are often called in the city or state government, and the positions generally are full-time. The CHWs typically are recruited for posts with specific programs, such as maternal health, asthma control, lead abatement, or cancer screening. The government agency provides them with training, usually disease or problem focused, matching the departmental structure within the agency. The agency is also responsible for monitoring and supervising the activities conducted by the CHWs, and they may use a variety of forms or meetings for this purpose, leading to the inevitable groans from CHWs about "paperwork." Well-known examples of programs where the CHWs are employed by a city or county agency are the Poder es Salud program in Portland, Oregon, and the Seattle-King County Healthy Homes program (see Table 5.1, column 3).

The advantages of being employed by a government agency are as follows:

- *Comprehensive training:* If the agency starts a program with CHWs, the agency generally develops a training program for them. The training programs developed and implemented by state or county governments are generally more complete, including 60–80 hours of training including the core competencies. Often taking advantage of funds and training models available from the Centers for Disease Control and Prevention (CDC), these training sessions are conducted by skilled trainers. These are particularly important for the immigrant CHWs whose written language skills may be limited. The training prepares the CHWs for a standardized protocol that is supported by the materials distributed at the training. Even when the agency funds the CHWs and they work offsite from the agency, they usually receive this training (McLearn et al., 2004). In Portland, Oregon, Multnomah County Health Department established a Community Capacitation Center, which developed an 80-hour curriculum based on the modules recommended by the National Health Advisor Study. In Oregon, any CHWs who have participated in this training program receive academic credit to be applied in other degree courses (Farquhar et al., 2008). A federally funded program, Healthy Families USA works through states in a similar way to provide standardized training to CHWs who work at local community organizations. This does not mean that the protocols are fixed permanently, as local groups may add to the activities to meet the needs of the families they see. In the case of Start Right, in order to address the very low vaccination coverage rates among immigrants in Washington Heights, three partners in the Healthy Families USA added training in promoting immunizations to the work they did with their families (Findley et al., 2006b).

• *Outreach across multiple communities:* When city and county agencies provide CHW services to address progressively their needs, they have a mandate to provide services for all residents, regardless of immigration status. Further, they are likely to work across multiple immigrant groups, and the county can bring them together to strengthen their solidarity and the development of stronger advocacy from a common base. In the case of Poder es Salud in Portland, Oregon, the county's Community Capacitation Center of Multnomah County brought together three different interest groups, and the CHWs working with each different interest group were able to learn from each other and the diverse groups: "Our dances may be different and our food may be different, but we're a lot alike. We share a whole lot, and we're going to help each other, because our communities are merging . . . it's good for us because it's going to be stronger" (Farquhar, Michael, and Wiggins, 2005). This type of inclusive and supportive environment for immigrants is more common in the more cosmopolitan regions of the country, and elsewhere much less likely.

• *Stable funding:* As employees of city or county government, these CHWs are regular employees of the agency and their positions are stable. Some federally funded programs offered by the CDC are generally available to state and county governments, and many CHW programs take advantage of these programs. Even if a program's funding is cut, it is possible for the agency to transfer the CHW from one program to another, thereby providing the CHW with employment security. Such transfers are also beneficial for the agency, because it facilitates the retention of a skilled CHW workforce (Peers for Progress, 2014).

• *Ties to community organizations and medical providers:* Several CHW programs involve CHWs who are employed by the county or city and do outreach and education, usually on selected issues, such as cancer screening or providing information about available maternal health services, as in Erie County, Ohio, or services targeting explicitly to deaf immigrants by the Hennepin County health department, Minnesota. In Seattle-King County, the health department teamed up with the public housing authority to identify and support families in public housing in addressing asthma triggers, following up with CHW visits to help families gain control of their children's asthma. CHWs were able to work with families speaking English, Spanish, or Vietnamese (Breysse et al., 2013; Krieger, Takaro, Song, and Wearver, 2005; Krieger et al., 2009). CHWs also may be assigned to work in specified communities with coalitions of providers and other community organizations, as in Prince George's County, Maryland, or Multnomah County, Oregon, where the Mexican immigrant CHWs working for the county worked through local churches (Farquhar et al., 2008; Wiggins et al., 2009). The East Harlem Asthma Center of Excellence is a program of the New York City Department of Health and Mental Hygiene, set up as a focal point where CHWs could link the community to physicians and other resources to gain control of asthma, a particular problem in this neighborhood. New York City also funded community organizations to hire CHWs to do outreach and education at hundreds of day care centers in neighborhoods with high rates of childhood asthma, and the city health department has recently established a Center for Health Equity which will have CHWs at the core of its operations. A good example of a county government supporting CHWs to improve links with providers while providing home visitation services is found in Seattle's King County (Krieger et al., 2005).

• *Career ladder, with training modules and standard supervision structure:* Within the civil service structure, it is possible to develop a career ladder for the CHWs, for example, public health advisor I, II, III (Farrar et al., 2011). Once there is a career ladder, this encourages the agency to develop stable training programs, as was the case in California where the City College of San Francisco developed a CHW certificate program (Love et al., 2004).

What are some of the disadvantages of having CHWs based at city or county government agencies?

- *Bureaucratic structure may reduce responsiveness:* Development of the protocols and procedures may take time, and once in place they may be slow to change, which might make the process difficult to be flexible in response to the needs of the immigrants.
- *Paperwork:* Government agencies often insist that CHWs complete multiple forms describing their activities, and this can become a burden.
- *Fear of government agencies:* Immigrants who lack documented status or those seeking to bring other family members are reluctant to openly obtain services from the government, even if they are freely available to them. They may still fear that participation will reduce their ability to sponsor others and/or lead the ICE agents to those they love. This is a major obstacle for many immigrants as their past experiences in their home countries have taught them that using government services can carry significant adverse consequences.
- *Vertical programs structure:* The vertical program structure that accompanies most agency budgeting and implementation isolates programs from each other. This vertical structure may restrict the ability of the CHW to respond comprehensively to the issues they discover in their work, and it may also mean they have less opportunity to share information with each other or to refer to each other's programs.
- *Top-down supervision:* The supervisors may be more concerned about "the numbers" than about CHW quality of service, and even if they are responsive to CHW questions, they may have little training in supportive supervision nor the CHW experience or skills to be able to appropriately support the CHWs.

In addition to these three basic models, there is a mixed model that combines the community-based CHW with some employment and program ownership from the government or health system, as in our own Asthma Basics for Children coalition, New York Presbyterian Hospital's WIN for Asthma, New York University's RICE program for Korean immigrants, La Red de Asma-Infantil in Puerto Rico, Starr County's border diabetes initiative, and Be Active Together in Seattle, Washington (see Table 5.1, column 4). A key feature of the mixed models is the sharing of responsibilities for training and supervising the CHWs between the health facility/agency and the community organizations. This is usually handled through a coalition structure in which the health facility and community partners are equal partners. For example, in the Asthma Basics for Children coalition, management decisions were made at a coalition level, while in WIN for Asthma, the management and supervision was done jointly by the hospital and specific CBO that employed the CHW (Peretz et al., 2012). This mixture achieves two key advantages of the facility-based and community-based models for institutional ownership of the CHW. The CHWs are based at the community partners with all the advantages of that model, but they also have a formally recognized role within the health system, which enhances their linkage to the medical care team. A similar structure exists in many maternal and child health CHW programs funded by health departments but supporting CHWs hired through community organizations.

- In the WIN for Asthma program, the CHWs rounded with the pediatric house staff, meeting potential participants for care coordination prior to discharge from the hospital, to tell them about the program when the parents were most aware of the importance of achieving control of their child's asthma. Once enrolled, however, the parents worked with the CHW at the community organization employing the CHW. Any problems juggling the CHW responsibilities between the hospital and the CBO were worked out by the two supervisors of that CHW. Any major problems that were found across two or more of the CBO partners were discussed and resolved by the coalition.
- In the case of Asthma Basics for Children, the hybrid resulted from the use of different models for employing CHWs in the program. Some worked for the hospital, some for CBOs, and a handful worked for schools. The coalition helped the supervisors across all these organizations in achieving a harmonization of responsibilities and expectations.
- In both the Seattle and Puerto Rico programs, the mixed model involved the city housing authorities, where the families live, the referral health facilities, and the community partners who hired and supported the CHWs. Coordination of supervision was handled through the coalition or partnership of the relevant agencies and organizations.

The mixed model also faces some challenges. Ideally, the CHWs are anchored in both the community and the health facility or governmental agency. Actually managing the mixed model requires both institutions to coordinate their activities with each other — no easy matter. Supervision issues can also arise, if the CHWs are supervised by one of the partners but not the other. In the WIN for Asthma model, the supervisors from the community organizations and the hospital met monthly to resolve any issues. They also jointly supervised the CHWs. Allocation of funds to support the CHWs can also be a tricky issue, if the partners cannot agree on appropriate separation of funding and supervision.

Which Elements of These Models Are Most Suitable for Work With Immigrants?

Our program reviews suggest that the most effective model for CHWs to support immigrant health is the mixed model, with funding coming from a large institutional source (health system or local government) but the home "base" for the CHWs to be in the community. With the opening of funding for CHWs in the United States under the Affordable Care Act, it is important for health systems to move quickly to fund CHW positions, but to do so in a way that allows the community partners to handle the recruitment and support of the CHWs. This combination of stable funding with community base is consistent with the decades old World Health Organization policy that stated: "Community health workers should be members of the communities where they work, should be selected by the communities, should be answerable to the communities for their activities, should be supported by the health system but not necessarily a part of its organization, and have shorter training than professional workers." (WHO, 1989, p. 6).

Being based in the community visibly demonstrates that the CHWs are by and for the community, and it facilitates the building of a trusting rapport that is the foundation for all they do to support immigrants. In the interviews conducted with CHWs working with immigrants, most CHWs advocated for retaining a stronger base in the community, at community organizations, with links to the hospital and health system. In addition to reaching immigrants who fear the system, this base reflects the more comprehensive assistance provided by CHWs, as compared to the medicalized version of case management offered by nurses at hospitals or large clinics. Here is how two CHW program managers articulated their preference for having CHWs based at community organizations:

> Currently, community-based organizations are facing a very big challenge with the medicalization of services. Case management by CHWs is now transferred to the hospital, with a focus on the medical aspect. Organizations lose resources, and the range of services they offer cannot be provided in the hospital setting. Also, by providing them in the hospital, we lose the

opportunity to empower CHWs to help each other. This will be bad for the services and for the community. Because case management is not just about taking medications, taking a piece of paper to the pharmacy, or monitoring adherence, the "enforcement" mindset. We need to keep our family-oriented, human approach, with emotional connections between the CHWs and the people. We need very flexible scheduling; we cannot be rigid. Can't do this in the hospital, even with the best intentions in the world. Hospitals are not society. They are completely different. You lose the balance and complementarity. Same budget, but won't be able to perform. Hospitals can't offer the same services. Sooner or later you will have to pay a price for that.

We need to strengthen community organizations. They are key to improving health and human services, particularly in New York. New York has so many people from so many different backgrounds, and this is what makes New York City New York. This needs to be reflected in the services provided. New York has to be creative in offering services from all types of agencies to address that diversity. In that sense, CHWs in the community-based organization are the adequate response.

Outreach and becoming known in the community is the base upon which all subsequent work with immigrants is based. CHWs reported that when they are coming from the immigrants' own church or favorite community organization, people felt that the CHW was meeting them on their home turf, easing the tensions they would normally feel toward an outsider trying to get them to go to the hospital. Immigrants fear coming to the hospital or to agencies for services, even if they qualify. In the words of one CHW working with the Dominican immigrants at one of the community organizations in Washington Heights:

To improve health care in the community we need to have people to go out into the community and advocate and let them know that they have nothing to fear, that they can come and get the services, and that we won't report them, and that it's free. Some services are free, but some of the families and some of the youth are not using the services that are available. Depending on the community that they are from, I think immigrants do use the services less than other people. As an example, if you're an immigrant and you speak English well, you know how to navigate the system a little better and you ask questions. If you don't speak the language, it's a barrier. So I think between immigrants, people who do speak English and those who don't, there is a barrier there between the ones who don't speak the language or the ones who don't know how to advocate for what they want are the ones who are left out.

While working for the health facilities conducting breast cancer screening, trained Southeast Asian CHWs worked through local Buddhist temples and churches to reach other Southeast Asian immigrants (Nguyen et al., 2011). This is how women who spoke with these CHW viewed their experience:

In my country, I never know what a Pap smear or mammogram is. . . . However, a navigator help me understand. Without the health navigator the conversation between the doctor and I will be fruitless. I am not able to describe my problems for him to help. . . . The health navigator provides me with mental and emotional support. They helped me feel confident and much less worried. The mental aspect, I think is very important.

And this is how the CHWs in this program viewed their experience:

From the CHW perspective, being in the community was viewed as very important for their success at reaching, engaging, and subsequently navigating the women through the health system. Because of their outreach to Buddhist temples and churches, the CHWs have built trusting relations between the sites and the health system. The providers in the system noted that the CHW had a pivotal role in linking the immigrants with their services, not just to get them there for screening but also to help with insurance and other supports. Builds confidence in the treatments. They helped the patient by providing them with access to information patients need to make the best decisions about their life.

When the CHWs are based in the community, this enormously facilitates empowerment. Hector Balcazar of the Salud para su Corazon program had this to say about the importance of community-based programs:

Within the context of a community-based program, the CHW model is a very real and promising strategy to help provide health-related service functions to the community in need. The CHW model has a unique quality for promoting the utilization of a variety of functional elements that help communities in need. Examples of functional elements include (1) unique engagement strategies with community members, with service units that can include community-based organizations, clinics, schools, and so on; (2) an elaborate process of dissemination of knowledge and practical information to members of the community; (3) a unique and well-balanced empowerment model that provides opportunities for community members to develop their potential as consumers of information and services and as human beings; and (4) a well-balanced approach to problem-solving strategies that community members can understand and respond to.

When CHWs are part of the community organization staff, such as a large multiservice community agency offering diverse services to address the wide array of problems immigrants experience, the CHW can easily make referrals to programs within the organization. Since the program is in-house, it is much easier for the CHW to follow up and make sure that the immigrant received the services, and similarly it is better for the immigrant, who trusts the CHW and his or her organization. Letty Guzman, the CHW supervisor of the Northern Manhattan Community Health Outreach Project (NOCHOP), had this to say about her work as an immigrant, working with other immigrants coming to Alianza Dominicana, the foremost community organization for Dominicans in New York City.

I am comfortable working in the community; I know the culture, the language. People are comfortable coming to a place they know. They can share, they can be open about what they eat; there are no barriers in expressing themselves. They can be honest about their issues. It would not be the same at a clinic; even if we were the same people, the hospital constrains people. They are afraid to express themselves to doctors and nurses. With a disease like diabetes, the greatest challenge is for people to break their habits. What we do is to help people change their habits. This does not start with the doctor. What we do that is different is that the change happens here. They can start here little by little, step by step, and when they hear from other participants, they can see that other people are also able to make changes. The participants also remind us that it is about their life, about health. It makes a big difference that this is here at Alianza, the organization they know and trust. Here at Alianza, we can offer many services here without referral out: Medicaid, housing (public

> housing applications, referral to shelters), food stamps, and immigration
> papers. People feel comfortable here at Alianza.

In a similar vein, Nadia Islam of New York University's CHW programs
spoke of the importance of the partnership of the medical center with community organizations. When looking for a partner who will be able to train
and support CHWs working with Asian immigrants, she said that they look
for partners with organizing experience, and those with relations to other
grassroots groups.

The community organizational base for CHWs also facilitates recruitment of immigrants who can be trained to become CHWs for their communities. Nadia Islam continued to highlight the advantages of this process of
recruitment, which is based on social networks, word of mouth, community
knowledge, and the personal attributes of trustworthiness and commitment
to helping other immigrants. Hector Balcazar commented that this recruitment through immigrant social networks has been very important for the
Salud para Su Corazon program.

> Over the last 5 or 10 years it has become easier to tap into existing CHW
> networks that have been created as a result of the increasing demand for hir-
> ing CHWs, even at part-time levels. More and more, there is greater clar-
> ity of intent to look for CHWs that have accumulated years of experience
> working in a variety of community programs. More and more, we have fewer
> problems identifying attributes we look for in CHWs we want to hire. This
> is a good sign for the CHW field and for CHWs who are so ready to enter
> the workforce.

Recruitment through immigrant social networks elicits CHWs who will then
network through these same social networks in their work promoting the
health of the immigrants. Jennifer Zanowiak, coordinator for the New York
University RICE program with Korean immigrants, commented on how
CHWs work through the community organization to achieve changes that
can only be made there:

> CHWs do not just dispense information. They make it a reality. They use
> their understanding of the community and knowledge of what works to
> develop activities for the community which recruit and retain people in the

program: walking tours, cooking demonstrations, picnics in the park, chess tournaments, and kite competitions. The CHWs pay attention to details because they want the participant experience with the CHW to be special. Through these activities in the community they provide information that is culturally meaningful and relevant for people. It is about seeking transformation and change, not just doing a task.

While it is not a given that the CHWs based at a community organization will have more flexibility in how they perform their tasks, the organizational context may lend itself to flexibility. In fact, such flexibility is needed for CHWs, regardless of where they work, as otherwise they cannot be responsive to the needs of the individual immigrants. In fact, if the county is mandated to provide given services to all persons, then it is the responsibility of the county to develop appropriate adaptations that will accommodate these differences, demonstrating system flexibility, not just flexibility for individual CHWs. As Nathan Ellis, director of Hennepin County (MN) Medical Center's Deaf and Immigrant Center for Education commented:

Say a hospital patient needs an X-ray, typically a procedure that is widely understood in American culture. No problem. But what if that patient is Russian, once lived near Chernobyl in the Ukraine, site of a terrible nuclear accident in the 1980s, and is terrified at the thought of radiation, plus that person not only does not speak English, but does not speak because he is deaf? Explaining becomes a major task. That "what-if" is a real-life example of the challenges facing Minnesota hospitals these days as staff encounter increasing numbers of immigrants, including deaf immigrants, thought to be about 10% of both general and immigrant populations. The story helps explain why Hennepin County Medical Center is expanding its services by opening the Deaf Immigrant Center for Education this week. Having a language barrier as well as hearing loss multiplies the challenges of explaining health information. CHWs in these programs tend to have a lot of flexibility in their work to provide whatever the client needs to be successful in understanding and managing their health and well-being. They are free to respond to the strengths and needs of the client.

As the Minnesota example illustrates, many hospitals have interpreter services to help patients who do not speak English, but these interpreter services seldom capture the full cultural nuances of the interchange between the provider and patient. Thus, in immigrant-friendly hospitals, CHWs are trained to work with patients, not just on translation of specific interchanges but on helping the patients to understand the system, their situation, their options, and, most important, to support them as they proceed in their care. What may work for the Korean immigrants may not work for the Somali immigrants, and CHWs need to be able to complement the translation with appropriate support to each immigrant group. We hear again from Nathan Ellis:

> The CHWs provide understanding of health, health promotion, disease prevention, and disease management; they are not just providing information itself. People who are immigrants face many challenges understanding our Western medical system and how to access services. They also have very different understanding of health and of the role of government. Fear of government and government services is widespread. There is also a broad fear that using services or disclosing illness will affect their application for residency or citizenship. For deaf and hard-of-hearing people, the situation is even more complicated because for them English is a second language. ASL [American Sign Language] is their first language. ASL is pretty good at transmitting information, but it is not very effective for promoting understanding. Because of this, people who use ASL have learned not to ask questions. They have also developed an experiential distrust that they will receive any answer to their question, or that the answer will be accurate. They typically will acquire information through ASL and then consult with a parent, partner, or close friend/relative to acquire understanding. If a deaf or hard-of-hearing person is an immigrant, then the challenge is confounded by the fact that English might be their third language, after their native language and ASL.

While community organizations tend to focus on one class of immigrants (e.g., Dominican, Southeast Asian, or African), large programs operated by hospitals and city and county government tend to have demands for service from multiple immigrant groups, such as in Hennepin County, where over 20 different languages need to be supported. Only large organizations have the human resource capacity to address such diverse populations. Thus, the ability to provide training and support to diverse immigrant populations is a major advantage of programs that hire or support CHWs through health facilities or governmental agencies. These programs have the resources needed to support development of basic training and coaching/health education materials in the primary language and then have them translated into the many languages spoken by immigrants in their community. The Community Capacitation Center of Multnomah County is an outstanding example of a comprehensive approach that supports the training of a diverse cadre of CHWs at community partners throughout the county. According to Noelle Wiggins, director of the program, an advantage of offering the training by the county is that the county bears the cost of developing the basic curriculum, materials, and trainers for "Poder es Salud," which can then be offered to multiple organizations. They are encouraged to tailor the training for the needs of specific immigrant groups. Because the training is a standardized package, graduates of the program receive a state certificate and are entered into the state CHW registry.

In New York, several hospitals and their partners have requested training from the CHW Network of New York City. Developed under the leadership of Sergio Matos, executive director of the CHW Network of NYC, the 70-hour training includes seven basic modules:

I: Essentials of Community Health Workers
II: Community Health Worker Empowerment Approach
III: Health Care Systems
IV: Community Health Worker Skills I—Outreach and Communication
V: Health Promotion and Behavior Change
VI: Community Health Worker Skills II—Counseling and Social Support
VII: Advocacy, Participatory Research, and Responsibility

Those requesting the training usually add 2–5 days of specialized training on the health issues that the CHWs are being asked to address (Matos et al., 2011; Ruiz et al., 2012). Several features of this curriculum are particularly critical for the training of immigrant CHWs or, more generally, CHWs for work with immigrant groups.

- Designed by and for CHWs (Catalani et al., 2009), and validated by rigorous research to assure that the curriculum covers skills that CHWs need and use for their work (Findley et al., 2012).
- Teaches evidence-based methods for CHWs to use in counseling and coaching families.

- Uses participatory or popular education methods of teaching, appropriate for adult learners and those with low literacy skills. This is particularly important for immigrant CHWs who may lack basic literacy skills in the national lingua franca or, for that matter, in any language.
- Training by CHW master trainers, consistent with evidence that shows that the most effective trainers are those who share the same roles and identities. Unlike many CHW training programs, the training is not offered by nurses or health educators, but by trainers prepared to use their own experience as a resource to inform their training. This training by master CHW trainers takes away the nervousness that immigrants may feel around academics and formal trainers and puts them at ease. When the CHW master trainers demonstrate how they solved problems or shared experiences with others when they were CHWs, the CHWs participating in the training can easily envision how they might use these skills themselves.
- Emphasis on empowering the CHWs to use their communication and coaching skills in a humanistic and dignified manner, respectful of the people with whom they are working and seeking in turn to empower them to become confident in making changes to their lives.
- Firmly frames the work of CHWs in a social justice context, using training processes that build solidarity among the CHWs and foster their self-esteem and self-perception as advocates for each other as well as for the community.

The network obtains feedback from all they have trained (well over 800), and it is uniformly positive, as the following comments illustrate:

> This program changes your heart, mind, and soul. It satisfied the craving to become a better person, not just a CHW. . . . This training helps you to look at oneself and clean up any problems. Then you can help others and that is something you need to do for a lifetime. . . . I wish the government would commission you to train all workers. I'm sad that just so few of us were exposed to you all.

The CHWs working for the New York University RICE and DREAM outreach projects were trained by the CHW Network of NYC, as were CHWs at the New York Presbyterian and Bronx-Lebanon Hospitals. Feedback from those trained at the New York University training showed that it built their confidence and their competence in critical cross-cultural communication skills, as well as providing them with the tools to be able to contextualize health education messages to their clients' situations (Ruiz et al., 2012). After taking the training, the CHW trainees, most of whom are immigrants themselves and some already working as CHWs, said:

> This training offers the hands-on, meaningful engagement that "knowledge" from books lacks. It enabled me to experience self-discovery, which I believe is the best way to learn and keep the knowledge always. The training has helped me to focus on the strengths of patients instead of being judgmental. We often do not realize the magnitude of the questions we ask clients, but this session really put me in the client's shoes. I feel I can now empower patients to advocate and learn to become independent in taking care of health. . . . The program also empowers us, the CHWs, and lights a fire within us.

The federal government is also involved in producing CHW training guides and materials, such as for the Diabetes Prevention Program of the CDC or Salud para su Corazon of the NIH/NHLBI, and these are also available to community organizations and public or private health providers. These training curricula are focused on particular diseases, however, and the organizations using them may still need to complement the disease-specific training with core competency training. Federal curricula, for example, may not be designed to be offered by CHWs, and this is a key feature of the CHW Network of NYC training. Further, they will need to adapt the training to the particular community's culture, language, and context, as was done with NOCHOP when it adapted the CDC "Small Steps, Big Rewards" for the Dominican community.

This shared training model is another recommended dimension of the mixed model we recommend for CHW programs working with immigrants. The CHWs are recruited, hired, and based at community organizations, but funding for hiring the CHWs comes from the larger institutional source (hospital or government), which also coordinates and supports the development of training and supporting materials for the CHWs. To avoid inappropriate and potentially culturally insensitive use of a national training materials, with this mixed model the training modules would need input from the community organizational partners and the CHWs themselves, to ensure that the resulting training is appropriate, meets recommendations for inclusion of core competency training, and uses an adult learning model that trains CHWs to coach and support the immigrants with whom they will work.

To have a lasting impact on how CHWs work, it is critical for the CHWs to have a clear job description summarizing their tasks, their mode of operation, and how they will be supervised and monitored. Many CHW programs have not paid a great deal of attention to the division of labor between the CHW and the other members of the health team, but this is very important for the CHW to be effective at bridging between the community and the health organization (Cherrington et al., 2008, 2010; Farquhar et al., 2008). In developing the CHW scope of practice for New York State, for example, the working group prepared a functional task analysis that identified exactly which activities were included in each core competency skill and how they would be monitored and supervised. For each of the core competency areas, there were 5–10 separate activities required to fulfill that competency.

Supervision is particularly important when the CHWs are working with immigrants of varying backgrounds and residency statuses. The leader of the Salud para du Corazon program in Texas, Hector Balcazar, pointed out:

> Supervision is another key topic that gradually is becoming a well-defined activity when CHWs are employed. In our experience, supervision, like in many other professions, has to be done with the highest level of integrity to give justice to the work CHWs do in many community projects. Like many human endeavors, a great supervisor makes for a great environment, and this environment facilitates the implementation of the CHW work. Unfortunately, I have seen in many instances where a poor supervisor is very detrimental to the work of CHWs. How many times CHWs are left behind in jobs without supervision and then blamed for their lack of adequate performance? This is not fair and we hope that as systems become more inclusive and democratic, we will see better supervision and integrity in the workforce environment for CHWs. On the other side of the spectrum, I have seen excellent supervisors take the highest level of integrity and action to guide CHWs to achieve the best they can bring to the job!

The solution in Poder es Salud and Bronx-Lebanon Family Medicine was to establish the principle that the CHWs would be supervised by a senior CHW, not by the nurse or medical practice director. In both the New York University and New York-Presbyterian mixed models, supervision is provided by a nonmedical person (public health or social work background), along with a supervisor from the community partner organization. This supervision provides CHWs with the support they need to distinguish personal versus professional boundaries with patients and to reinforce the underlying scope of work and practice guidelines for the CHWs. Ideally, this supervision is interactive, and involves direct observation of the CHW providing counsel and coaching to community members. Feedback to the New York University program suggests that there is agreement that this supervision needs to be one on one, provided in communities where the CHWs are working, and facilitate problem resolution.

In the WIN for Asthma program at New York-Presbyterian Hospital, supervision was provided jointly by the program manager at the community organization and the program manager at the hospital, and in no case from the nursing or medical staff (Peretz et al., 2012). This was a win-win all the way around for the participants, CHWs, community organizations, and the health care providers. One of the CHWs said, "I'm very happy with my supervision. Something that you need is to be confident with the people who are around you, and I'm receiving that from my supervisor and other staff members." Her supervisor and the health care provider in the clinic all reported being pleased with the support that the CHW was providing to families. They all agreed that the work with families at the community organization and escorting patients on the visits to the doctor were key elements in helping families open up and begin to appropriately manage their child's asthma.

Conclusions

Programs working with immigrants need a high degree of trust and community presence, yet the CHWs in these programs also need to be prepared for a wide range of problems, not just health, but legal, housing, employment, and educational. The most appropriate organizational model appears to be a mixed model, with the CHWs based at community organizations.

To be fully empowered within the community, they need to be very closely affiliated with the community organization, as an employee or associate, full-time or part-time. This provides the CHW with the opening toe hold into the immigrant community, and it invests the CHW with the credibility and trust that is already felt for this organization. Senior CHWs at the organization can provide mentoring and supervision to the CHWs recruited for specific programs.

To make the connections with the health facility and particularly to truly bridge between the immigrants and the health facility, the mixed model is advantageous. While the CHW may be employed or at least seconded to the community organization, if the CHW is also employed or given status within the health facility, this will provide the channels through which the CHW can connect immigrants to the health facility. Consistent with the patient-centered medical home, the mixed model would assign to the CHW a specific role within the medical team and a recognized status with providers, who will accept the CHW as an advocate and supporter for the immigrant patients. Because the health facility may work with multiple immigrant groups, the mixed model allows the facility to partner with different community organizations reaching out into different immigrant groups.

The health facility is likely to have the resources to support development of a more comprehensive training for the CHWs. However, advocating for the mixed model does not mean that the training needs to be conducted by nurses, and a major advantage of the mixed model is that it provides a framework to ensure collaboration between the community organization, CHWs, and the health facility in developing the protocol and training for the CHWs. The health facility has an interest in following state or national guidelines for core competency training, as this will facilitate certification of the CHWs so that they can be reimbursed through available channels, while the community organization has an interest in ensuring that the training is empowering and gives the CHWs the skills they need to be able to help immigrants change their lives.

Though the CHWs may be employed by the community organization, the best supervisory model is likely to be similar to that used by WIN for Asthma, with joint supervision by the community organization and the health facility. The facility, particularly a large hospital or network, is likely to have social workers and a full complement of services of value to immigrants: counseling, insurance enrollers, and referrals for legal aid.

For immigrant health programs focusing on prevention, where consultations with medical providers are not a large part of the work, the mixed model can be a partnership between the community organizations and the city or county. In this case, the city or county would be the funder and provider of comprehensive training for the CHWs, potentially also providing other materials supporting the work of the CHWs. Programs also could take advantage of city or county programs addressing immigrant needs, for example, housing or legal aid.

While it may be more complicated to implement a mixed model, the mixed model also provides a more solid base for the development, implementation, and sustainability of immigrant health programs with CHWs. The examples presented in this chapter show that the patience and attention to detail needed to implement mixed models are well rewarded. These programs appear well positioned to address multiple needs of immigrants, at the same time that they are also well positioned to transition into sustainable, permanent programs making the facility or government agency immigrant friendly and open to diverse populations.

6

Strengthening the Bridge: How We Can Support Community Health Workers in Their Work With Immigrants

ALMOST DAILY, THE newspapers of the world cover stories about immigrants: children riding the rails from Central America to "El Norte," Syrians fleeing into Turkey, whole boatloads of African immigrants drowning, sometimes at the hands of their captains, as they attempt to cross over to Spain or Italy, Muslims fleeing persecution in Myanmar, Liberian children in Texas being shunned due to irrational fears of Ebola, young Tunisians having stones thrown at them as they attempt to scale a border fence in Italy, Ukrainians fleeing conflict, and so on. While these stories aim to help us better understand the human side of the immigration process, the overwhelming message that uninformed readers get is one of distress, that the immigrant situation poses huge problems which we are ill equipped to solve. We have written this book as an antidote to that "too big to solve" mantra. Yes, the problems are huge, but no, they are not hopeless. Immigrant health issues can be addressed, to the benefit of the immigrants and their communities, and community health workers (CHWs) are central to the strategy to do this in a humane and effective fashion. In this concluding chapter, we summarize the lessons we have gleaned in our journey, making recommendations for integrating CHWs into our strategies for supporting immigrants to become and stay healthy as they make their way in the world.

Better Integrate Immigrants Into Our Societies

Worldwide, roughly 2.5 million men, women, and children leave their home countries to make a life for themselves elsewhere. Over half settle in the upper-income countries of the "North," and the remainder settle in the low- and middle-income countries lumped together as the "South." The majority of the world's international immigrants head for the cities, which are their ports of entry or poles of attraction with both large immigrant communities providing shelter to subsequent arrivals and the hubs of the largest and most diverse labor markets. One in five international migrants heads for one of twenty metropolitan areas in nine nations, each now having 1 million or more immigrants, and cities with at least 100,000 immigrants are scattered across the United States, Canada. and Europe, as well as a handful in Australia, Asia, Latin America, and the Middle East. Immigrant neighborhoods flourish in cities throughout the world (Price and Benton-Short, 2008).

Over one third (40%) of the world's immigrants head to the United States, which receives about 1 million legal immigrants per year, and the number of undocumented immigrants may reach as high as 800,000 per year (Meissner, Meyers, Papademitriou, and Fix, 2006; United Nations Department of Economic and Social Affairs, 2011). Although the United States continues to absorb this enormous volume of immigrants, it is doing so with mixed feelings. After years of high unemployment rates and ever-mounting fears of terrorism, the Statue of Liberty image of the nation welcoming the sick and the poor is no longer one shared by all. The melting-pot image of the United States has become tarnished, as politicians in national and state legislatures pander to the xenophobic fears of many Americans towards immigrants with attempts at ever more exclusionary regulations, tacit support for the deportation of thousands of undocumented immigrants, and failure to provide humane and reasonable supports for immigrant families, as would have been possible with the failed immigration reform bill which would have prevented deportation of some parents of child immigrants.

The United States is not alone in seeking to fence out immigrants, and most nations have tightened their restrictions on immigration. As here in the United States, most of these efforts are not effective, as immigrants are exceptionally creative and able to move despite walls or "closed borders." Indeed, we benefit from more open borders. Contrary to popular fears that immigrants take away jobs from the native-born, the evidence presented in Chapter 1 suggests that the immigrants play a vital role in filling entry-level and low-wage positions that native-born Americans do not want but that actually contribute to upward mobility for the rest of the labor force. Our economies benefit from the influx of skilled labor when professionals move from one country to the next. Immigrants are well represented among the innovators whose ideas are driving economic growth in new sectors. Further, the fears that immigrants take from the system more than they pay in are completely unfounded; in fact, immigrants pay more in taxes than they take out as benefits to themselves or their families (Meissner et al., 2006; United Nations Department of Economic and Social Affairs, 2013).

It is time to recognize that we need and benefit from international migrants, and our policies should endeavor to rationalize the flows so that the potential power of immigrant contributions is facilitated, not thwarted. There needs to be more flexibility in the types of immigration visas, including more temporary and transitional visas, allowing in more total legal immigrants. We also need practical and humane pathways to citizenship/residency for the millions of undocumented immigrants living in our communities and contributing to our economy. We especially need to protect children born or raised in this country from having their parents taken away and deported. Breaking up families has never before been a part of the American ethos. Enforcement of existing immigration regulations needs to be made more humane and less chaotic, so that families do not live in perpetual fear of deportation of one or more of their members. Greater clarity about immigration status and rights can reduce fear and help more individuals be willing to trust that the system is there to help them, not to catch and hurt them.

Expand Health Care Access for Immigrants

In 2008, the United Nations adopted a resolution on the health of migrants, calling for equitable access to services and migrant-sensitive health policies. This resolution specifically identified the need to build the capacity of health service providers to reach out to and address the health needs of immigrants (World Health Organization, 2011). As discussed in Chapter 1, a significant handicap that immigrants face in addressing their health issues is that many do not have health insurance. Further, among those with insurance or access to free health care, accessing and using the health care system is problematic. In the United States, many immigrants who are eligible for health insurance through their employer or through Medicaid/Medicare do not obtain insurance.

In the United States, the passage of the Affordable Care Act means that millions of legal immigrants can now obtain coverage, but as yet they have been slow to enroll, including in New York, despite a strong immigrant advocacy group, the New York Immigration Coalition (Vimo & Weiner, 2013). We heard from immigrants and CHWs alike that they need help in overcoming the administrative hurdles in applying for and using health insurance. We agree with the New York Immigration Coalition recommendations promoting "one-stop services" to enable mixed-status families to apply through one portal for the different insurance products for which they are eligible, as well as with several other steps to facilitate insurance applications by immigrants through the New York Exchange. The coalition also recommends that community organizations apply for Affordable Care Act funds to hire CHWs—navigators—to assist immigrants with enrollments, on both the main exchange and the small business exchange.

Make Health Promotion Immigrant-Friendly

But simply obtaining insurance is not enough, and immigrants unfamiliar with the health system or with how health insurance works need help in understanding when and how to use this insurance to pay for services. Just as obtaining insurance requires a patient navigator to help the immigrant understand the different options, immigrants need help using their insurance, in communicating to the clerks, nurses, and physicians they will encounter, and in knowing what to do with the prescriptions and other recommendations they receive from these providers. While we have focused on the problems of immigrants in the United States, such difficulties are not unique to the United States and have been experienced by immigrants in a variety of European cities.

Immigrants need more than a translation service. In their home countries, health is not just freedom from disease. Health is larger than that; it is having enough to eat and being able to show that you are living a good life. As we discussed in Chapter 1, immigrants are eager to adopt the ways of their new community, for example, to have their children attend the local schools and learn English, to find work, and to find a home and settle down. They want to be proud of their achievements, and one way to do this is to take their children to McDonalds for Big Macs or to buy a television so their children can watch cartoons like all the other children. Yet, fast food and watching television contribute to overweight and a host of related health problems. Who will tell the immigrant families that their proud actions might not be good in the long run? If they hear this message on the radio or see it on a billboard on the subway, they may not understand or pay attention. What is needed are personal interventions, akin to the navigator in the health system, someone in the community—a CHW—who will help the immigrants to understand how the much vaunted McDonalds may not be a good choice and to find other ways to demonstrate their progress in becoming part of mainstream society. And for those who are struggling to put any food on the table, the CHW can point the way to food pantries or soup kitchens and help them sign up for WIC or other food benefits.

Support Immigrants with Community Health Workers

The health system is designed to "fix" problems, namely to provide medicine and other medical interventions that cure acute illness episodes. For immigrants with little or no familiarity with hospitals or clinical care, this is both bewildering and alien. They need someone to translate the care recommendations into language and concepts they understand. Evidence presented in Chapter 2 shows that CHWs fill this need extremely well, explaining the care recommendations and facilitating culturally appropriate communication between the health provider and the immigrant. They are the bridge between the immigrant and the alien world of the health system.

However, the role of the CHW is perhaps more important outside the system. As noted in Chapter 2, much of health happens at home and in the community. CHWs understand that health means different things to different people. If people are hungry, then the CHW understands that the family needs food and sends them to a food pantry. If the family is facing eviction, the CHW understands that shelter and security are the primary concerns, and helps them get legal aid to fight eviction. The CHW understands that to speak to someone about asthma medications when he or she has much bigger worries is a waste of everyone's time, and the CHW knows to shape his or her support according to the family priorities, not some fixed agenda. When the CHW has demonstrated that the family's welfare comes first, then the family will trust the CHW and be willing to listen to health messages from the CHW. As we showed in Chapter 3 on becoming a CHW, the CHW needs both humility to accept the person-centered priorities plus sensitivity and skill to be able to communicate complicated health messages in a language and methods that the immigrants can understand.

This mutual understanding and respect is the fundamental basis for empowerment. The CHW becomes empowered to advocate for and support the efforts of the immigrants in seeking health care from the hospital or clinic. Outside the health system and in the community, the CHW supports the broader empowerment of the immigrant to solve fundamental survival issues and to take charge of their health. CHWs are part of the mindset for reclaiming our own responsibility for staying healthy. Thus, the CHW is the two-way bridge, ideally facilitating changes in the health system that make it more immigrant friendly and remove inequitable barriers to care. At the same time, the CHW facilitates a reframing of how immigrants understand "health" and opens up a vision of choices immigrants can make to actively steer their families along a pathway to long-term health and well-being.

Nurture Immigrants to Become Community Health Workers

Immigrants who become CHWs have the experience and passion to serve other immigrant families, and we recommend that priority be given to nurturing immigrants to become CHWs. As discussed in Chapter 3, becoming a CHW takes passion and commitment. To be a CHW is to be a master of multitasking, an artful communicator, a creative educator, a thoughtful and sensitive counselor, a thorough worker leaving no stone unturned, and one who is persistent in the face of multiple obstacles. This is arduous work that requires the individual to dig down deep inside to be able to give sincerely from the heart.

Immigrants who want to become CHWs have repeatedly demonstrated that they have this passion, energy, and commitment. As immigrants themselves, they have experienced the trauma of leaving home and the long, grueling, and sometimes perilous voyage to their new home. They drew on enormous inner strengths to make this voyage, and then continued to use this strength to overcome the many obstacles and hardships endured while becoming settled. Out of the pain of this experience they developed a passion to help others get over these hurdles, hopefully with less difficulty and anguish than they endured. Like a phoenix rising from the ashes, immigrants who become CHWs have the potential to become very powerful advocates and supporters for other fellow travelers.

The immigrant who becomes a CHW is also the most welcome among other immigrants. When the CHW who is also an immigrant approaches other immigrants, it is as if the CHW were already part of the immigrant's family, and he or she is welcomed. In this context, the CHW empowerment activities with the family are akin to a 12-step program, with the CHW using his own experience, strength and hope to propose steps that he has already taken himself, and then supporting the immigrants as they progressively take more and more responsibility for themselves.

Arelia, the immigrant from Peru introduced in the first chapter, became a CHW, and her story illustrates brilliantly how that immigrant experience shaped her vision of being a CHW.

From day one I have been becoming a CHW, I guess because I was inspired that my parents had been CHWs in Peru. Ever since I came, I have been helping people at my church in the neighborhood and at the soup kitchen. Because I had to learn these things myself, I could explain to people where to go to solve problems; I helped them understand what was going on with them. I actually became a CHW because of my nephew's asthma. My sister and her son had been living with me since he was born. He started having breathing problems when he was 2. The doctors gave us a bunch of medications, and my father and I wanted to follow the doctor's advice and give the medicines, while my mom believed in home remedies, Matthew was very sick, so we did everything the doctor said. Then, I gave him too many "pumps" because I just wanted him to stop coughing, so he "overdosed" (began trembling and got panicky), so we had to take him to the emergency room. It was hard for me to grasp what was happening. I needed to learn about the disease, go to the library to use the computer, so I could ask the doctor questions. I kept thinking: Why did I have to work so hard to find answers? Why didn't the doctor answer my questions? My sister did not have papers so it was scary for her to go to the doctor. What I was really wanting was someone who could help me figure out what to do for my nephew. That is when I realized that I could be that person. So, at the library I learned all about asthma, and gradually I learned how to control it better. I am self-taught on becoming a CHW; I assembled all the resources. I learned a lot about the health system from friendly faces, people who want to help you, in the library, where they mention a lot about services. Many of the friendly faces I met turned out to be CHWs I met at the clinic. I did not know it then, but I now realize they were. The CHWs were also immigrants. They spoke Spanish and English with an accent. All Latinas. So, I knew that they were immigrants and I could tell them about me, because I could see me in them. I could be honest that I did not have documentation. I knew they would understand me because they were Latina, too.

My first job as a CHW was as an outreach worker at Safe Space, a community-based multi-service agency, to help families use the services, including family asthma programs. I had the answers to all their questions. When they closed out their community asthma program, I went to work for a health plan, still providing asthma education and support to immigrant families. Then, I went to work for a multiservice agency as a CHW, in an asthma initiative linked to Woodhull Hospital. I learned so much more about asthma from working with Dr. Fishkin, and he soon asked me to be the supervisor for the program. Even though I didn't have the credentials, I learned and was able to be promoted. I was better at my job than some people who have an MA! Now I am the supervisor for the CHW program in Family Medicine at the Bronx-Lebanon Hospital. In fact, they want to promote me again, but I am happy. I have my dream. I am a CHW. I went back to school at night and earned my AA degree and then finally my Bachelor of Arts degree in 2014. I am working at a major hospital, and I love my work.

Being an immigrant, I could understand their issues, living it. I didn't have to judge them if they had or did not have papers. And this helped me to talk with them without fear. When they heard my story, I shared my story, I connected with them. I could really ask about their dreams, their hopes, and the main point is that I could understand about how their immigrant issues affected what they could or did do to control asthma. The social issues were the biggest concerns for people, and this made control difficult. My greatest satisfaction now is when I can see the progression in families from day one to the end of the year, that they are getting on top of their social issues, and then they are ready and willing to deal with asthma. It is as if they say, "OK, Arelia, you helped me with my issues, now I will help you with 'your' asthma issues." They still want to take their home remedies, like my mom, but every family became a success. They ended up doing what they needed to do and we celebrated it. It was big for them and big for me, too. It was small on the way, but big in the end.

I am always thinking about my mom's reaction to the health care system here when we came. She was asking, "Why we can't just go to get health care? Why if we have no papers are we treated as second-class citizens?" From my own experience, I think CHWs should be in every facility, to give advice to the immigrant families, especially the undocumented. If we had CHWs everywhere, this would be a big help for the immigrant community. To guide immigrants is huge. The problems are hard to solve, but we have to get started.

As Arelia demonstrates so well through her experiences, immigrant CHWs are adept at interpersonal communication and coaching, going far beyond simple language translation to facilitating truly cross-cultural communication. They can explain health care recommendations in ways that the immigrants understand and can follow. More important, in a society where immigrants are fearful of the system and anyone who might lead to troubles with immigration, the immigrant CHW is trusted and welcomed to their home as others would not be. Once the immigrant CHW becomes trusted, the immigrant CHW has credibility in both worlds and can serve as a bidirectional bridge between the home and the health system.

Locate Community Health Worker Programs in Immigrant Communities

Effective CHW programs are community-driven and community-oriented, integrating health promotion activities into the heart of community educational and social service institutions. As shared in Chapter 4, our experience with the Northern Manhattan health promotion coalitions underscores the importance of structuring the immigrant health program with a very strong base in the community. The strategies for how to promote recommended health behaviors were developed with community input and tailored carefully to the particular needs of the immigrant families. The CHWs worked by and for the community partners, and they were responsive to the community, continually adapting their programs to families' needs. Throughout the coalitions, there was a sense that the CHWs were working for the people, not for the "system," and this sense of ownership facilitated the positive response we experienced throughout the community.

In addition, the coalitions were able to fully embrace the CHW strategy, because they were given multiple options for how to mobilize CHWs. They could choose to have volunteer or paid CHWs, full-time or part-time, and, importantly, staff who became CHWs by virtue of additional training and support for coalition health-related activities. Most chose to add CHW roles to the work responsibilities of existing staff, for example, day care providers or family support workers in parenting programs, and they saw this as a "win–win" enhancing their staff capacity to support families without having to add another layer of workers. Where the organizations engaged volunteer CHWs, they were in no way denigrated as "only" volunteers. Each organization and each individual CHW's choice was respected, and the contributions of all CHWs were integrated into the overall work of the coalition.

We used a variety of strategies to fund their work, including full-time or part-time salaries, casual wages for days worked, and incentives or bonuses for high performance. As shown in Chapter 4, only a minority were full-time salaried CHWs paid entirely from the coalition's grants or by hospital partners. The limited resources were stretched by cost-sharing with partner organizations, whereby the coalition grant and the organization shared the cost of a CHW's salary. In other cases, the CHWs were part-time; some paid regularly, some paid per day worked. All had opportunities for performance bonuses when they exceeded performance expectations. This creative funding enabled many more CHWs, over 2,500, to be trained and mobilized, than if the coalition had to pay for 100% of their salaries.

With the CHWs based in community organizations, day care programs, schools, and faith-based organizations throughout the community, they had incredible reach into the immigrant community, contacting almost 170,000 persons over the decade of operation. Because the CHWs had multiple opportunities to personally interact with the families they contacted, they were able to turn interest into participation for a very large number of families who were eligible for the coalition's services, about half of all those eligible.

The CHWs also were successful at reaching and engaging immigrant families, because most were immigrants themselves. They used their immigrant experience to gain the trust of families and to demonstrate possibilities for change. When CHWs spoke of doing outreach in the community, they were talking about walking in their own neighborhoods, among people who came to know and respect them for their work. The coalition also made sure that these immigrant CHWs were properly oriented and trained to engage and support their neighbors, gradually enabling them to grasp and act on the health care recommendations.

The last critical element contributing to the success of the coalitions was the partnership with community health care providers. The coalition ensured that the health care providers at all the community's clinics were aware of the coalitions, trained in multicultural communication, and willing to go the extra mile to care for immigrant patients. We wanted to make sure that the doctors would be ready to respond when we mobilized immigrants to ask questions during their visits with the doctor. However, we also made it clear that the community groups were leading the coalition, not the health care providers. This made it possible for CHWs to "bridge the gap" on their own terms, linking the families to the providers in a gradual process that built trust in the providers.

Partner to support Immigrant Health Programs

In Chapter 5 we saw that programs working with immigrants need a high degree of trust and community presence, and the most appropriate organizational model appears to be a mixed partnership model, with the CHWs based at community organizations, but with strong links to health care organizations or local governments to support training and referrals. This provides CHWs with the opening toe hold into the immigrant community, and it invests the CHWs with the credibility and trust that is already felt for this organization. Based in the community, the CHW can be maximally responsive to the broad range of needs of immigrants and able to support community advocacy for housing, food, schools, day care, workforce equity, and other basic issues vital to reducing the suffering and vulnerability of immigrants.

In order to address immigrants' health needs and to connect them to the health facility, the mixed or partnership model is advantageous. The mixed model gives the CHW credibility in the health system or local agency, thereby facilitating the bridging their work. With this stature, the CHW is well positioned to help the immigrant communicate with the facility and navigate the system to obtain the services needed. This is particularly important for immigrants with chronic diseases or multiple chronic diseases requiring numerous visits with varied providers. Another advantage of the mixed model is that the health facility is likely to have the resources to support development of a more comprehensive training for the CHWs. With the mixed partnership model, a central training institute can provide training to multiple immigrant health programs, with the institute supported by contributions from stakeholders, including major health plan partners or the state. Caution is needed, however, to avoid overspecializing the CHWs and thereby jeopardizing their holistic health approach.

Expand CHW Programs for Immigrants Globally

The partnership model of CHWs promoting the health of immigrants is applicable worldwide, but it is primarily needed in the 100+ metropolitan areas where immigrants tend to concentrate. While much of this book has focused on the ways that CHWs promote the health of immigrants in the United States, we believe that this model will work well in other countries. The 1978 United Nations Alma Ata declaration of "Health for All" and the more recent 2008 "Health for Migrants" declarations provide the rationale for immigrant health programs. A close reading of the 1978 Alma Ata declaration points almost directly to CHWs as the key strategy to achieve health for all. As outlined in the declaration, "Health for All" does not mean an end to disease and disability, nor that doctors and nurses will care for everyone. Health begins at home, and it is reinforced in schools, at work, and in daily living (Bassett, 2006). Health is protected when people take charge of staying healthy and shaping their lives to be free from the burden of disease. Most interpretations of Alma Ata have focused on its call for universal primary health care and an equitable distribution of health resources, but these miss the vital role of health promotion within the community. If we are to apply the Alma Ata declaration to immigrants, it directly points to the need for CHWs to work within immigrant communities to help them take charge of their health and reduce inequities in accessing and using available health care resources.

As noted in Chapter 2, the global profile and activities of CHWs are similar to that found in the United States, and just as immigrants become passionate about becoming CHWs in New York, there are likely to be immigrants in Toronto, London, Paris, or Hong Kong who will want to work with their fellow immigrants. The process of recruiting and training the immigrants to work in global settings may differ slightly from that found in the United States. One of the key differences may be that in many countries, health systems often have a niche for CHWs within the health system, which tends to be filled by native-born graduates of the CHW training institutes. If immigrant CHWs are to be recruited, the organizations and agencies seeking to launch a program will have to directly recruit CHWs from among the relevant immigrant population. Some may already have trained or worked as a CHW prior to arrival, like Arelia's parents, but if not, additional training will be needed. As in the United States, we recommend that the training include the same basic core competency skills as were recommended for immigrant CHWs in the United States.

Although globally more CHWs work in rural than urban areas, it is likely that the greatest need for the immigrant health programs will be in the largest cities of the world, as this is where immigrants are increasingly concentrating. As of 2005, 102 cities worldwide were home to 100,000 or more international migrants (Price and Benton-Short, 2008). While the United States still dominates as the country with the most cities with large immigrant populations, cities with large immigrant populations are located throughout Europe and the Middle East, as well as in Asia, Latin America, and Africa. Immigrants in these cities face similar problems to those identified in the United States, and we believe that the recommendations we have made for CHWs to promote the health of immigrants in the United States are equally valid for other countries. As in the United States, the greatest areas of health needs for immigrants to these large cities are likely to be very similar to those found in the United States: maternal health care, infant and child health, chronic disease prevention and management, and mental health issues.

As in the United States, there are likely to be a variety of organizational structures within which CHWs can work to promote immigrant health, but the principle of basing the immigrant CHW in the community is still the preferred model, for all the same reasons as in the United States. Immigrants everywhere tend to shy away from the "system," particularly if they are not formally registered as a resident or do not have work papers. CHWs living and working in the immigrant enclaves will have a much greater chance of being accepted, trusted, and effective. It is also likely that programs will use a variety of staffing patterns to obtain the requisite complement of CHWs. In Canada and Europe, there are parenting programs comparable to the Healthy Families USA and Head Start programs. These programs could do the same thing we did in New York City, where we trained family support workers in health promotion so they could become CHWs, incorporating the CHW tasks into their ongoing work. Some may be recruited as volunteers or part-timers, and, as in the United States, programs will likely need to be creative in developing funding strategies for the CHWs.

These CHWs working at local community organizations also can benefit from the partnership or mixed model of organizational structure. With this model, training and related supports are provided through a local government agency, large health center, or a specialized health worker training institute. European educational systems tend to provide a wider range of certificates, and often these are free to the students, who may even receive a stipend to support their living costs during training. Ideally, a specialized health training institute would be able to develop and offer an appropriate adaptation of the Community Health Extension Worker training common in Anglophone Africa, but tailored for CHWs working with immigrants in an urban setting. As was recommended for the mixed model in the United States, the curriculum would need to have add-ons for multicultural communication and immigrant-specific content, including advocacy for nonhealth issues.

Millions of immigrants could benefit from well-crafted CHW programs. As they benefit, the world will benefit. This is a challenge we can ill afford to ignore. The challenge is great, but it is not insurmountable. As Arelia said, "The problems are hard to solve, but we have the pieces." The CHWs have the will; immigrants have the need. If we want "Health for All," we need CHWs to be on the frontlines advocating for them and supporting them in their struggle to live well in all senses of the word.

References

Abraido-Lanza, A.F., M.T. Chao, and K.R. Florez. 2005. Do healthy behaviors decline with greater acculturation? Implications for the Latino mortality paradox. *Social Science and Medicine, 61*(6), 1243–1255.

Abraido-Lanza, A.F., B.P. Dohrenwend, D.S. Ng-Mak, and J.B. Turner. 1999. The Latino mortality paradox: A test of the "salmon bias" and healthy migrant hypotheses. *American Journal of Public Health, 89*(10), 1543.

Acevedo-Garcia, D., M.J. Soobade R, and L.F. Berkman. 2007. Low birthweight among US Hispanic/Latino subgroups: The effect of maternal foreign-born status and education. *Social Science and Medicine, 65*(12), 2503–2516.

Ackerman, R., E. Finch, E. Brizendine, H. Zhou, and D. Marrero. 2008. Translating the diabetes prevention program into the community: The DEPLOY pilot study. *American Journal of Preventive Medicine, 35*(4), 357–363.

Ackermann, R.T. 2013. Working with the YMCA to implement the diabetes prevention program. *American Journal of Preventive Medicine, 44*(4, Supplement 4), S352–S356.

Adair, R., J. Christianson, D.R. Wholey, K. White, R. Town, S. Lee, . . . D. Elumba. 2012. Care guides: Employing nonclinical laypersons to help primary care teams manage chronic disease. *Journal of Ambulatory Care Management, 35*(1), 27–37.

Adler, N.E., and J.M. Ostrove. 1999. Socioeconomic status and health: What we know and what we don't. *Annals of the New York Academy of Science, 896*, 3–15.

Akresh, I.R., and R. Frank. 2008. Health selection among new immigrants. *American Journal of Public Health, 98*(11), 2058–2064.

Albright, A.L., and E.W. Gregg. 2013. Preventing type 2 diabetes in communities across the U.S.: The National Diabetes Prevention Program. *American Journal of Preventive Medicine, 44*(4, Supplement 4), S346–S351.

Ali, M.K., J.B. Echouffo-Tcheugui, and D.F. Williamson. 2012. How effective were lifestyle interventions in real-world settings that were modeled on the diabetes prevention program? *Health Affairs, 31*(1), 67–75.

Allen, J.K., C.R.D. Himmelfarb, S.L. Szanton, L. Bone, M.N. Hill, and D.M. Levine. 2011. COACH trial: A randomized controlled trial of nurse practitioner/community health worker cardiovascular disease risk reduction in urban community health centers: Rationale and design. *Contemporary Clinical Trials, 32*(3), 403–411.

Antecol, H., and K. Bedard. 2006. Unhealthy assimilation: Why do immigrants converge to American health status levels? *Demography, 43*(2), 337–360.

Argeseanu Cunningham, S., J.D. Ruben, and K.M. Narayan. 2008. Health of foreign-born people in the United States: A review. *Health Place, 14*(4), 623–635.

Babamoto, K.S., K.A. Sey, A.J. Camilleri, V.J. Karlan, J. Catalasan, and D.E. Morisky. 2009. Improving diabetes care and health measures among Hispanics using community health workers: Results from a randomized controlled trial. *Health Education and Behavior, 36*(1), 113–126.

Baker, M.K., K. Simpson, B. Lloyd, A.E. Bauman, and M.A.F. Singh. 2011. Behavioral strategies in diabetes prevention programs: A systematic review of randomized controlled trials. *Diabetes Research and Clinical Practice, 91*(1), 1–12.

Balcázar, H. 2009. A Promotora de Salud model for addressing cardiovascular disease risk factors in the US-Mexico border region. *Preventing Chronic Disease, 6*(1), A02.

Balcazar, H. 2011. Salud para su Corazon (Health for your Heart) community health worker model: Community and clinical approaches for addressing cardiovascular disease risk reduction in Hispanics/Latinos. *Journal of Ambulatory Care Management, 34*(4), 362–372.

Balcazar, H., E.L. Rosenthal, J.N. Brownstein, C.H. Rush, S. Matos, and L. Hernandez. 2011. Community health workers can be a public health force for change in the United States: Three actions for a new paradigm. *American Journal of Public Health, 101*(12), 2199–2203.

Balcazar, H.G., T.L. Byrd, M. Ortiz, S.R. Tondapu, and M. Chavez. 2009. A randomized community intervention to improve hypertension control among Mexican Americans: Using the Promotoras de Salud community outreach model. *Journal of Health Care for the Poor and Underserved, 20*(4), 1079–1094.

Baquero, B., G.X. Ayala, E.M. Arredondo, N.R. Campbell, D.J. Slymen, L. Gallo, and J.P. Elder. 2009. Secretos de la Buena Vida: Processes of dietary change via a tailored nutrition communication intervention for Latinas. *Health Education Research, 24*(5), 855–866.

Bassett, M.T. 2006. Health for all in the 21st century. *American Journal of Public Health, 96*(12), 2089.

Batalova, J., and A. Lee. 2014. Frequently requested statistics on immigrants and immigration in the United States. *Migration Policy Institute.* Retrieved December 2014, from http://www.migrationpolicy.org/article/frequently-requested-statistics-immigrants-and-immigration-united-states

Battaglia, T., L. McCloskey, S. Caron, S. Murrell, E. Bernstein, A. Childs, ... J. Bernstein. 2012. Feasibility of chronic disease patient navigation in an urban primary care practice. *Journal of Ambulatory Care and Management, 35*(1), 38–49.

Berkman, L.F., and S.L. Syme. 1979. Social networks, host resistance, and mortality: A nine-year follow-up study of Alameda County residents. *American Journal of Epidemiology, 109*(2), 186–204.

Bhutta, Z., Z.S. Lassi, G. Pariyo, and L. Huicho. 2010. *Global experience of community health workers for delivery of health-related millennium development goals: A systematic review, country case studies, and recommendations for integration into national health systems.* Global Health Workforce Alliance. Geneva, Switzerland: World Health Organization.

Bhutta, Z.A., J.K. Das, N. Walker, A. Rizvi, H. Campbell, I. Rudan, and R.E. Black. 2013. Interventions to address deaths from childhood pneumonia and diarrhoea equitably: What works and at what cost? *The Lancet, 381*(9875), 1417–1429.

Borrell, L.N., and E.A. Lancet. 2012. Race/ethnicity and all-cause mortality in US adults: Revisiting the Hispanic paradox. *American Journal of Public Health, 102*(5), 836–843.

Breysse, J., S. Dixon, J. Gregory, M. Philby, D.E. Jacobs, and J. Krieger. 2013. Effect of weatherization combined with community health worker in-home education on asthma control. *American Journal of Public Health, 104*(1), e57–e64.

Brown, H., K. Wilson, J. Pagan, C. Arcari, M. Martinez, K. Smith, and B. Reininger. 2012. Cost-effectiveness analysis of a community health worker intervention for low-income Hispanic adults with diabetes. *Preventing Chronic Disease, 9*(12), 1–9.

Brown, S., A. Garcia, and K. Kouzekanani. 2002. Culturally competent diabetes self-management education for Mexican Americans: The Starr County border health initiative. *Diabetes Care, 25*(2), 259–268.

Brownson, C.A., T.J. Hoerger, E.B. Fisher, and K.E. Kilpatrick. 2009. Cost-effectiveness of diabetes self-management programs in community primary-care settings. *Diabetes Educator, 35*(5), 761–769.

Brownstein, J.N., L.R. Bone, C.R. Dennison, M.N. Hill, M.T. Kim, and D.M. Levine. 2005. Community health workers as interventionists in the prevention and control of heart disease and stroke. *American Journal of Preventive Medicine, 29*(5, Supplement 1), 128–133.

Bryant-Stephens, T., C. Kurian, R. Guo, and H. Zhao. 2009. Impact of a household environmental intervention delivered by lay health workers on asthma symptom control in urban, disadvantaged children with asthma. *American Journal of Public Health, 99*(Supplement 3), S657–S665.

Bryant-Stephens, T., and Y. Li. 2008. Outcomes of a home-based environmental remediation for urban children with asthma. *Journal of the National Medical Association, 100*(3), 306–316.

Buttenheim, A., N. Goldman, A.R. Pebley, R. Wong, and C. Chung. 2010. Do Mexican immigrants "import" social gradients in health to the US? *Social Science and Medicine, 71*(7), 1268–1276.

Caban, A., and E.A. Walker. 2006. A systematic review of research on culturally relevant issues for Hispanics with diabetes. *Diabetes Educator, 32*(4), 584–595.

Calderon, J., M. Bazargan, N. Sangasubana, R. Hays, P. Hardigan, and R. Baker. 2010. A comparison of two educational methods on immigrant breast cancer knowledge and screening behaviors. *Journal of Health Care for the Poor and Underserved, 21*(1), 76–90.

Cantril, C., and P.J. Haylock. 2013. Patient navigation in the oncology care setting. *Seminars in Oncology Nursing, 29*(2), 76–90.

Capps, R., and M. Fix. 2013. Immigration reform: A long road to citizenship and insurance coverage. *Health Affairs (Millwood), 32*(4), 639–642.

Capps, R., M. Rosenblum, and M. Fix. 2009. *Immigrants and health care reform: What's really at stake?* Washington, DC: Migration Policy Institute.

Castles, S. 2000. International migration at the beginning of the twenty-first century: Global trends and issues. *International Social Science Journal, 52*(3), 269–281.

Castles, S. 2002. Migration and community formation under conditions of globalization. *International Migration Review, 36*(4), 1143–1168.

Catalani, C.E., S.E. Findley, S. Matos, and R. Rodriguez. 2009. Community health worker insights on their training and certification. *Progress in Community Health Partnerships, 3*(3), 201–202.

Cherrington, A., G.X. Ayala, H. Amick, J. Allison, G. Corbie-Smith, and I. Scarinci. 2008. Implementing the community health worker model within diabetes management: Challenges and lessons learned from programs across the United States. *Diabetes Educator, 34*(5), 824–833.

Cherrington, A., G.X. Ayala, J.P. Elder, E.M. Arredondo, M. Fouad, and I. Scarinci. 2010. Recognizing the diverse roles of community health workers in the elmination of health disparities: From paid staff to volunteers. *Ethnicity and Disease, 20*, 189–194.

Cordasco, K.M., N.A. Ponce, M.S. Gatchell, B. Traudt, and J.J. Escarce. 2011. English language proficiency and geographical proximity to a safety net clinic as a predictor of health care access. *Journal of Immigrant and Minority Health, 13*(2), 260–267.

Corkery, E., C. Palmer, M.E. Foley, C.B. Schechter, L. Fisher, and S.H. Roman. 1997. Effect of a bicultural community health worker on completion of diabetes education in a Hispanic population. *Diabetes Care, 20*, 254–257.

Cornell, C.E., M.A. Littleton, P.G. Greene, L. Pulley, J.N. Brownstein, B.K. Sanderson, . . . J.M. Raczynski. 2009. A community health advisor program to reduce cardiovascular risk among rural African-American women. *Health Education Research, 24*(4), 622–633.

Coughey, K., G. Klein, C. West, J.J. Diamond, A. Santana, E. McCarville, and M.P. Rosenthal. 2010. The Child Asthma Link Line: A coalition-initiated, telephone-based, care coordination intervention for childhood asthma. *Journal of Asthma, 47*(3), 303–309.

Culica, D., J.W. Walton, K. Harker, and E.A. Prezio. 2008. Effectiveness of a community health worker as sole diabetes educator: Comparison of CoDE with similar culturally appropriate interventions. *Journal of Health Care for the Poor and Underserved, 19*(4), 1076–1095.

Derose, K.P., J.J. Escarce, and N. Lurie. 2007. Immigrants and health care: Sources of vulnerability. *Health Affairs, 26*(5), 1258–1268.

DiNapoli, T.P., and K. Bleiwas. 2008. *An economic snapshot of Washington Heights and Inwood.* New York, NY: New York City Public Information Office.

Drieling, R.L., J. Ma, and R.S. Stafford. 2011. Evaluating clinic and community-based lifestyle interventions for obesity reduction in a low-income Latino neighborhood: Vivamos Activos Fair Oaks Program. *BMC Public Health, 11,* 98.

Druss, B.G., L. Zhao, S.A. von Esenwein, J.R. Bona, L. Fricks, S. Jenkins-Tucker, . . . K. Lorig. 2010. The Health and Recovery Peer (HARP) Program: A peer-led intervention to improve medical self-management for persons with serious mental illness. *Schizophrenia Research, 118*(1–3), 264–270.

Edberg, M., S. Cleary, and A. Vyas. 2010. A trajectory model for understanding and assessing health disparities in immigrant/refugee communities. *Journal of Immigrant and Minority Health, 13,* 576–584.

Elo, I.T., Z. Vang, and J.F. Culhane. 2014. Variation in birth outcomes by mother's country of birth among non-Hispanic Black women in the United States. *Maternal and Child Health Journal, 18*(10), 2371–2381.

Fagman, L.J., D.A. Dorr, M. Davis, P. McGinnis, J. Mahler, M.M. King, and L. Michaels. 2011. Turning on the care coordination switch in rural primary care: Voices from the practices—Clinician champions, clinician partners, administrators, and nurse care managers. *Journal of Ambulatory Care and Management, 34*(3), 304–318.

Farquhar, S.A., and Y.L. Michael. 2004. Poder es Salud/Power for Health: An application of the community health worker model in Portland, Oregon. *Journal of Interprofessional Care, 18*(4), 445–447.

Farquhar, S.A., Y.L. Michael, and N. Wiggins. 2005. Building on leadership and social capital to create change in 2 urban communities. *American Journal of Public Health, 95*(4), 596–601.

Farquhar, S.A., N. Wiggins, Y.L. Michael, G. Luhr, J. Jordan, and A. Lopez. 2008. "Sitting in different chairs:" Roles of the community health workers in the Poder es Salud/Power for Health Project. *Education for Health (Abingdon), 21*(2), 39.

Farrar, B., J.C. Morgan, E. Chuang, and T.R. Konrad. 2011. Growing your own: Communithy health workers and jobs to careers. *Journal of Ambulatory Care and Management, 34*(3), 234–246.

Fernandes, R., K. Braun, J. Spinner, C. Sturdevant, S. Ancheta, S. Yoshimura, ... C. Lee. 2012. Healthy Heart, Healthy Family: A NHLBI/HRSA collaborative employing community health workers to improve heart health. *Journal of Health Care for the Poor and Underserved, 23,* 988–999.

Fernandez, M.E., A. Gonzales, G. Tortolero-Luna, J. Williams, M. Saavedra-Embesi, W. Chan, and S.W. Vernon. 2009. Effectiveness of Cultivando la Salud: A breast and cervical cancer screening promotion program for low-income Hispanic women. *American Journal of Public Health, 99*(5), 936–943.

Finch, B.K., and W.A. Vega. 2003. Acculturation stress, social support, and self-rated health among Latinos in California. *Journal of Immigrant and Minority Health*, *5*(3), 109–117.

Findley, S., S. Matos, A. Hicks, A. Campbell, A. Moore, and D. Diaz. 2012. Building a consensus on CHW scope of practice: Lessons from New York. *American Journal of Public Health, 102*(10), 1981–1987.

Findley, S., M. Rosenthal, T. Bryant-Stephens, M. Damitz, M. Lara, C. Mansfield, ... M. Viswanathan. 2011. Community-based care coordination: Practical applications for childhood asthma. *Health Promotion Practice, 12*(6 Supplement 1), 52S–62S.

Findley, S.E. 2001. Compelled to move: The rise of forced migration in sub-Saharan Africa. In M. Siddique (Ed.), *International migration into the 21st century* (pp. 275–310). Cheltenham, UK & Northampton, MA: Edward Elgar.

Findley, S.E., M. Irigoyen, M. Sanchez, L. Guzman, M. Mejia, M. Sajous, ... F. Chimkin. 2006a. Community-based strategies to promote childhood immunizations. *Health Promotion Practice, 7*(S3), 191S–200S.

Findley, S.E., M. Irigoyen, M. Sanchez, L. Guzman, M. Mejia, ... F. Chimkin. 2006b. Community-based strategies to reduce childhood immunization disparities. *Health Promotion Practice, 7*(3 Supplement), 191S–200S.

Findley, S.E., S. Matos, A. Hicks, J. Chang, and D. Reich. 2014. Community health worker integration into the health care team accomplishes the triple aim in a patient-centered medical home. *Journal of Ambulatory Care and Management, 37*(1), 82–91.

Findley, S.E., G. Thomas, R. Madera-Reese, N. McLeod, S. Kintala, R. Andres-Martinez, ... E. Herman. 2011. A community-based strategy for improving asthma management and outcomes for preschoolers. *Journal of Urban Health*, 88(Supplement 1), 85–99.

Finucane, M.L., and C.K. McMullen. 2008. Making diabetes self-management education culturally relevant for Filipino Americans in Hawaii. *Diabetes Educator, 34*(5), 841–853.

Fisher-Owens, S.A., G. Boddupalli, and S.M. Thyne. 2011. Telephone case management for asthma: An acceptable and effective intervention within a diverse pediatric population. *Journal of Asthma, 48*(2), 156–161.

Fleury, J., C. Keller, A. Perez, and S. Lee. 2009. The role of lay health advisors in cardiovascular risk reduction: A review. *American Journal of Community Psychology, 44*(1–2), 28–42.

Formicola, A., and L. Hernandez-Cordero. 2012. *Mobilizing the community for better health: What the rest of America can learn from Northern Manhattan.* New York, NY: Columbia University Press.

Formicola, A., M. Perez, and J. McIntosh. 2012. Creating the collaborative foundation. In A. Formicola and L. Hernandez-Cordero (Eds.), *Mobilizing the community for better health: What the rest of America can learn from Northern Manhattan* (pp. 14–24). New York, NY: Columbia University Press

Fox, P., P.G. Porter, S.H. Lob, J.H. Boer, D.A. Rocha, and J.W. Adelson. 2007. Improving asthma-related health outcomes among low-income, multiethnic, school-aged children: Results of a demonstration project that combined continuous quality improvement and community health worker strategies. *Pediatrics*, *120*(4), e902–e911.

Freeman, H.P. 2013. The history, principles, and future of patient navigation: Commentary. *Seminars in Oncology Nursing*, *29*(2), 72–75.

Freire, P. 1970. *Pedagogy of the oppressed*. New York, NY: Seabury Press.

Friedman, A.R., F.D. Butterfoss, J.W. Krieger, J.W. Peterson, M. Dwyer, K. Wicklund, . . . L. Smith. 2006. Allies community health workers: Bridging the gap. *Health Promotion Practice*, *7*(2 Supplement), 96S–107S.

Fronek, P., M. Kendall, G. Ungerer, J. Malt, E. Eugarde, and T. Geraghty. 2009. Towards healthy professional-client relationships: The value of an interprofessional training course. *Journal of Interprofessional Care*, *23*(1), 16–29.

Fujiwara, T., and M.H. Chan. 2009. Role of behavioral outreach worker in increasing mental health service utilization for children. *Pediatrics International*, *51*(1), 167–168.

Gadd, M., J. Sundquist, S.E. Johansson, and P. Wandell. 2005. Do immigrants have an increased prevalence of unhealthy behaviours and risk factors for coronary heart disease? *European Journal of Cardiovascular Prevention and Rehabilitation*, *12*(6), 535–541.

Gany, F., A. Levy, P. Basu, and S. Misra. 2012. Culturally tailored health camps and cardiovascular risk among South Asian immigrants. *Journal of Health Care for the Poor and Underserved*, *23*(2), 615–625.

Garcia, C., D. Hermann, A. Bartels, P. Matamoros, L. Dick-Olson, and J. Guerra de Patino. 2012. Development of Project Wings home visits: A mental health intervention for Latino families using community-based participatory research. *Health Promotion Practice*, *13*(6), 755–762.

Gawande, A. 2011, January 24. The hot spotters: Can we lower medical costs by giving the neediest patients better care? *The New Yorker*, 1–10.

Getaneh, A., W. Michelen, and S. Findley. 2008 The prevalence of cardiovascular risk conditions and awareness among a Latino sub-group: Dominicans in Northern Manhattan. *Ethnicity and Disease*, Spring. *18*, 342–347.

Goldman, N., R.T. Kimbro, C.M. Turra, and A.R. Pebley. 2006. Socioeconomic gradients in health for White and Mexican-origin populations. *American Journal of Public Health*, *96*(12), 2186–2193.

Green, L.W., and M.W. Kreuter. 1999. *Health promotion planning: An educational and ecological approach*. Mountain View, CA: Mayfield Publishing.

Grigg-Saito, D., R. Toof, L. Silka, S. Liang, L. Sou, L. Najarian, . . . S. Och. 2010. Long-term development of a "whole community" best practice model to address health disparities in the Cambodian refugee and immigrant community of Lowell, Massachusetts. *American Journal of Public Health*, *100*, 2026–2029.

Guendelman, S., V. Angulo, M. Wier, and D. Oman. 2005. Overcoming the odds: Access to care for immigrant children in working poor families in California. *Maternal and Child Health Journal*, *9*(4), 351–362.

Guendelman, S., H.H. Schauffler, and M. Pearl. 2001. Unfriendly shores: How immigrant children fare in the U.S. health system. *Health Affairs (Millwood)*, *20*(1), 257–266.

Guendelman, S., D. Thornton, J. Gould, and N. Hosang. 2006. Mexican women in California: Differentials in maternal morbidity between foreign and US-born populations. *Paediatrica and Perinatal Epidemiology*, *20*(6), 471–481.

Gushulak, B.D., and D.W. Macpherson. 2006. The basic principles of migration health: Population mobility and gaps in disease prevalence. *Emerging Themes in Epidemiology*, *3*, 3.

Gusmano, M.K. 2012. Undocumented immigrants in the United States: Use of health care. Hastings Center Issue Brief, March 27, 2012, pp. 1–6. Garrison, NY: The Hastings Center.

Hagan, J., N. Rodriguez, R. Capps, and N. Kabiri. 2003. The effects of recent welfare and immigration reforms on immigrants' access to health care. *International Migration Review*, *37*(2), 444.

Han, H.R., K.B. Kim, and M.T. Kim. 2007. Evaluation of the training of Korean community health workers for chronic disease management. *Health Education Research*, *22*(4), 513–521.

Hargraves, J.L., W. Ferguson, C. Lemay, and J. Pernice. 2012. Community health workers assisting patients with diabetes in self-management. *Journal of Ambulatory Care and Management*, *35*(1), 15–26.

Harvey, I., A. Schulz, B. Israel, S. Sand, D. Myric, M. Lockett, . . . Y. Hill. 2009. The Healthy Connections Project: A community-based participatory research project involving women at risk for diabetes and hypertension. *Progress in Community Health Partnerships*, *3*(4), 273–274.

Hatton, T., and J. Williamson. 2011. Are Third World emigration forces abating? *World Development*, *39*, 20–32.

Hawkins, D., and D. Groves. 2011. The future role of community health centers in a changing health care landscape. *Journal of Ambulatory Care and Management*, *34*(1), 90–99.

Heisler, M., M. Spencer, J. Forman, C. Robinson, C. Shultz, G. Palmisano, . . . E. Kieffer. 2009. Participants' assessments of the effects of a community health worker intervention on their diabetes self-management and interactions with healthcare providers. *American Journal of Preventive Medicine*, *37*(6 Supplement 1), S270–S279.

Herman, A.A. 2011. Community health workers and integrated primary care teams in the 21st century. *Journal of Ambulatory Care and Management*, *34*(4), 354–361.

Hill, N., E. Hunt, and K. Hyrkäs. 2012. Somali immigrant women's health care experiences and beliefs regarding pregnancy and birth in the United States. *Journal of Transcultural Nursing*, 23(1), 72–81.

Horowitz, C.R., K.A. Colson, P.L. Hebert, and K. Lancaster. 2004. Barriers to buying healthy foods for people with diabetes: Evidence of environmental disparities. *American Journal of Public Health*, 94(9), 1549–1554.

Horowitz, C.R., L. Tuzzio, M. Rojas, S.A. Monteith, and J.E. Sisk. 2004. How do urban African Americans and Latinos view the influence of diet on hypertension? *Journal Health Care Poor Underserved*, 15(4), 631–644.

Huang, G., and J. London. 2012. Mapping cumulative environmental effects, social vulnerability, and health in the San Joaquin Valley, California. *American Journal of Public Health*, 102(5), 830–832.

Hummer, R.A., D.A. Powers, S.G. Pullum, G.L. Gossman, and W.P. Frisbie. 2007. Paradox found (again): Infant mortality among the Mexican-origin population in the United States. *Demography*, 44(3), 441–457.

Hunter, J.B., J.G. de Zapien, M. Papenfuss, M.L. Fernandez, J. Meister, and A.R. Giuliano. 2004. The impact of a Promotora on increasing routine chronic disease prevention among women aged 40 and older at the U.S.-Mexico border. *Health Education and Behavior*, 31(4 Supplement), 18S–28S.

Ingram, M., G. Gallegos, and J. Elenes. 2005. Diabetes is a community issue: The critical elements of a successful outreach and education model on the U.S.-Mexico border. *Preventing Chronic Disease*, 2(1), A15.

Islam, N., J. Zanowiak, L. Wyatt, K. Chun, L. Lee, S. Kwon, and C. Trinh-Shevrin. 2013. A randomized-controlled, pilot intervention on diabetes prevention and healthy lifestyles in the New York City Korean community. *Journal of Community Health*, 38(6), 1030–1041.

Jasso, G., D.S. Massey, M.R. Rosenzweig, and J.P. Smith. 2004. Immigrant health: Selectivity and acculturation. Presented at *National Conference on Racial and Ethnic Disparities in Health* (pp. 1–48). Baltimore, MD: National Academy of Sciences.

Joshu, C.E., L. Rangel, O. Garcia, C.A. Brownson, and M.L. O'Toole. 2007. Integration of a Promotora-led self-management program into a system of care. *Diabetes Educator*, 33(Supplement_6), 151S–158S.

Kahssay, H., M. Taylor, and P. Berman. 1998. *Community health workers: The way forward*. Geneva, Switzerland: World Health Organization.

Kangovi, S., N. Mitra, D. Grande, M.L. White, S. McCollum, J. Sellman,. . . J. Long. 2014. Patient-centered community health worker intervention to improve post-hospital outcomes: A randomized clinical trial. *JAMA Internal Medicine*, 174(4), 535–543.

Katula, J.A., M.Z. Vitolins, T.M. Morgan, M.S. Lawlor, C.S. Blackwell, S.P. Isom, ... D.C. Goff, Jr. 2013. The Healthy Living Partnerships to Prevent Diabetes

Study: Two-year outcomes of a randomized controlled trial. *American Journal of Preventive Medicine, 44*(4, Supplement 4), S324–S332.

Katula, J.A., M.Z. Vitolins, E.L. Rosenberger, C.S. Blackwell, T.M. Morgan, M.S. Lawlor, and J.D.C. Goff. 2011. One-year results of a community-based translation of the Diabetes Prevention Program: Healthy-Living Partnerships to Prevent Diabetes (HELP PD) project. *Diabetes Care, 34*(7), 1451–1457.

Kaushal, N. 2009. Adversities of acculturation? Prevalence of obesity among immigrants. *Health Economics, 18*(3), 291–303.

Keller, T., W.J. Borges, M.M. Hoke, and T. Radasa. 2011. Promotores and the chronic care model: An organizational assessment. *Journal of Community Health Nursing, 28*(1), 70–80.

Krieger, J., T.K. Takaro, L. Song, N. Beaudet, and K. Edwards. 2009. A randomized controlled trial of asthma self-management support comparing clinic-based nurses and in-home community health workers: The Seattle-King County Healthy Homes II Project. *Archives of Pediatric and Adolescent Medicine, 163*(2), 141–149.

Krieger, J.W., T.K. Takaro, L. Song, and M. Weaver. 2005. The Seattle-King County Healthy Homes Project: A randomized, controlled trial of a community health worker intervention to decrease exposure to indoor asthma triggers. *American Journal of Public Health, 95*(4), 652–659.

Krieger, N., A. Kosheleva, P.D. Waterman, J.T. Chen, and K. Koenen. 2011. Racial discrimination, psychological distress, and self-rated health among US-born and foreign-born Black Americans. *American Journal of Public Health, 101*(9), 1704–1713.

Lara, M., L. Akinbami, G. Flores, and H. Morgenstern. 2006. Heterogeneity of childhood asthma among Hispanic children: Puerto Rican children bear a disproportionate burden. *Pediatrics, 117*(1), 43–53.

Lara, M., C. Gamboa, M.I. Kahramanian, L.S. Morales, and D.E. Bautista. 2005. Acculturation and Latino health in the United States: A review of the literature and its sociopolitical context. *Annual Review of Public Health, 26*, 367–397.

Lara, M., G. Ramos-Valencia, J. Gonzales-Gavillan, F. Lopez-Malpica, B. Morales-Reyes, H. Marin, ... H. Mitchell. 2013. Reducing quality-of-care disparities in childhood asthma: La Red de Asma Infantil intervention in San Juan, Puerto Rico. *Pediatrics, 131*(S1), S26–S37.

Lara, M., G.R. Valencia, J.A. Gavillan, B.M. Reyes, C. Arabia, F.L. Malpica, ... M. Chinman. 2009. Reducing inequities among children with asthma in the island of Puerto Rico: Experiences of a community-based, trans-sectoral effort. *Journal Health Care for the Poor and Underserved, 20*(4 Supplement), 116–136.

Lasser, K.E., D.U. Himmelstein, and S. Woolhandler. 2006. Access to care, health status and health disparities in the United States and Canada: Results of a cross-national population-based survey. *American Journal of of Public Health, 96*(7), 1300–1307.

Lassetter, J., and L. Callister. 2009. The impact of migration on the health of voluntary migrants in western societies. *Journal of Transcultural Nursing, 20,* 93–104.

Lassi, Z.S., A. Majeed, S. Rashid, M.Y. Yakoob, and Z.A. Bhutta. 2013. The interconnections between maternal and newborn health—evidence and implications for policy. *Journal of Maternal-Fetal and Neonatal Medicine, 26*(S1), 3–53.

Lehmann, U., and D. Sanders. 2007. *Community health workers: What do we know about them?* Evidence and Information for Policy Technical Brief, Dept. of Human Resources for Health. Geneva, Switzerland: World Health Organization.

Lewin, S., S. Munabi-Babigumira, C. Glenton, K. Daniels, X. Bosch-Capblanch, B.E. van Wyk, . . . I.B. Scheel. 2010. Lay healthworkers in primary and community health care for maternal and child health and the management of infectious diseases (Review). *The Cochrane Library,* (3), 1–173.

Li, V., P. Goethals, and S. Dorfman. 2008. A global review of training of community health workers. *International Quarterly of Community Health Education, 27*(3), 181–218.

Litwin, H. 2010. Social networks and well-being: A comparison of older people in Mediterranean and non-Mediterranean countries. *Journal Gerontology B: Psychological Sciences and Social Sciences, 65*(5), 599–608.

Lob, S.H., J.H. Boer, P.G. Porter, D. Núñez, and P. Fox. 2011. Promoting best-care practices in childhood asthma: Quality improvement in community health centers. *Pediatrics, 128*(1), 20–28.

Lobo, A.P., and J.J. Salvo. 2013. *The newest New Yorkers: Characteristics of the city's foreign-born population.* New York City Department of City Planning. New York, NY: New York City.

Lopez-Acuna, D. 2010. *Health of migrants-the way forward: Report of a global consultation. Madrid, Spain 3–5 March 2010.* Geneva, Switzerland: World Health Organization.

Lorig, K., P. Ritter, F. Villa, and J. Armas. 2009. Community-based peer-led diabetes self-management: A randomized trial. *Diabetes Educator, 35*(4), 641–651.

Lorig, K., P. Ritter, F.J. Villa, and J.D. Piette. 2008. Spanish diabetes self-management with and without automated telephone reinforcement. *Diabetes Care, 31,* 408–414.

Lorig, K.R., P.L. Ritter, and A. Jacquez. 2005. Outcomes of border health Spanish/English chronic disease self-management programs. *Diabetes Educator, 31*(3), 401–409.

Loucks, E.B., L.M. Sullivan, R.B. D'Agostino, Sr., M.G. Larson, L.F. Berkman, and E.J. Benjamin. 2006. Social networks and inflammatory markers in the Framingham Heart Study. *Journal of Biosocial Science, 38*(6), 835–842.

Love, M.B., V. Legion, J.K. Shim, C. Tsai, V. Quijano, and C. Davis. 2004. CHWs get credit: A 10-year history of the first college-credit certificate for community health workers in the United States. *Health Promotion Practice, 5*(4), 418–428.

Lujan, J., S.K. Ostwald, and M. Ortiz. 2007. Promotora diabetes intervention for Mexican Americans. *Diabetes Educator, 33*(4), 660–670.

Macintyre, S., A. Ellaway, R. Hiscock, A. Kearns, G. Der, and L. McKay. 2003. What features of the home and the area might help to explain observed relationships between housing tenure and health? Evidence from the west of Scotland. *Health and Place, 9*(3), 207–218.

Mainous, A.G., 3rd, V.A. Diaz, and M.E. Geesey. 2008. Acculturation and healthy lifestyle among Latinos with diabetes. *Annals of Family Medicine, 6*(2), 131–137.

Margellos-Anast, H., M.A. Gutierrez, and S. Whitman. 2012. Improving asthma management among African-American children via a community health worker model: Findings from a Chicago-based pilot intervention. *Journal of Asthma, 49*(4), 380–389.

Markova, T., M. Mateo, and L.M. Roth. 2012. Implementing teams in a patient-centered medical home residency practice: Lessons learned. *Journal of the American Board of Family Medicine, 25,* 224–231.

Marsiglia, F., M. Bermudez-Parsai, and D. Coonrod. 2010. Familias Sanas: An intervention designed to increase rates of postpartum visits among Latinas. *Journal of Health Care for the Poor and Underserved, 21,* 119–131.

Martin, M.A., G.S. Mosnaim, D. Rojas, O. Hernandez, and L.S. Sadowski. 2011. Evaluation of an asthma medication training program for immigrant Mexican community health workers. *Progress in Community Health Partnerships, 5*(1), 95–103.

Martin, P., and E. Midgeley. 2010. *Immigration in America 2010.* Population Bulletin Update. Washington, DC: Population Reference Bureau.

Martinez Garcel, J. 2012. Casting an A-team to deliver results: Embedding and sustaining the role of community health workers in medical homes. *Medical Home News, 4*(2), 6–7.

Martinez, J., M. Ro, N. W. Villa, W. Powell, and J.R. Knickman. 2011. Transforming the delivery of care in the post–health reform era: What role will community health workers play? *American Journal of Public Health, 101*(12), e1–e5.

Massey, D. 2006. Patterns and processes of international migration in the 21st century: Lessons for South Africa. In M. Tienda, S. Findley, S. Tollman, and E. Preston-Whyte (Eds.), *Africans on the move: African migration and urbanization in comparative perspective* (pp. 38–70). Johannesburg, South Africa: University of Wittswatersrand Press.

Massey, D.S. 1990. Social structure, household strategies, and the cumulative causation of migration. *Population Index, 56*(1), 3–26.

Massey, D.S. 2002. Thinking the unthinkable: The immigration myth exposed. *Population and Development Review, 28*(2), 358–360.

Matos, S., S.E. Findley, A. Hicks, and L. Do Canto. 2011. *Paving a path to advance the community health worker workforce in New York State: A new summary report and recommendations.* New York, NY: Community Health Worker Network of

NYC, New York State Health Foundation, Columbia University Mailman School of Public Health.

May, M.L., and R.B. Contreras. 2007. Promotor(a)s, the organizations in which they work, and an emerging paradox: How organizational structure and scope impact promotor(a)s' work. *Health Policy, 82*(2), 153–166.

McClure, H.H., J.J. Snodgrass, C.R. Martinez, Jr., J.M. Eddy, R.A. Jimenez, and L.E. Isiordia. 2010. Discrimination, psychosocial stress, and health among Latin American immigrants in Oregon. *American Journal of Human Biology, 22*(3), 421–423.

McLearn, K.T., D.M. Strobino, C.S. Minkovitz, E. Marks, D. Bishai, and W. Hou. 2004. Narrowing the income gaps in preventive care for young children: Families in Healthy Steps. *Journal of Urban Health, 81*(4), 556–567.

Meghea, C.I., B. Li, Q. Zhu, J.E. Raffo, J.K. Lindsay, J.S. Moore, and L.A. Roman. 2013. Infant health effects of a nurse–community health worker home visitation programme: A randomized controlled trial. *Child: Care, Health and Development, 39*(1), 27–35.

Meissner, D., D.W. Meyers, D.G. Papademitriou, and M. Fix. 2006. Immigration and America's future: A new chapter. *Report of the Independent Task Force on Immigration and America's Future* (pp. 1–42). New York, NY: Migration Policy Institute.

Messias, D., D. Parra-Medina, P. Sharpe, L. Trevino, A. Koskan, and D. Morales-Campos. 2013. Promotoras de salud: Roles, responsibiltes and contributions in a multisite community-based randomized controlled trial. *Hispanic Health Care International, 11*(2), 62–71.

Michael, Y.L., S.A. Farquhar, N. Wiggins, and M.K. Green. 2008. Findings from a community-based participatory prevention research intervention designed to increase social capital in Latino and African American communities. *Journal of Immigrant and Minority Health, 10*, 281–289.

Minkler, M., A.P. Garcia, J. Williams, T. LoPresti, and J. Lilly. 2010. Si se Puede: Using participatory research to promote environmental justice in a Latino community in San Diego, California. *Journal of Urban Health, 87*(5), 796–812.

Mitchell, E.A., P.B. Didsbury, N. Kruithof, E. Robinson, M. Milmine, M. Barry, and J. Newman. 2005. A randomized controlled trial of an asthma clinical pathway for children in general practice. *Acta Paediatrica, 94*(2), 226–233.

Mock, J., S.J. McPhee, T. Nguyen, C. Wong, H. Doan, K.Q. Lai, . . . N. Bui-Tong. 2007. Effective lay health worker outreach and media-based education for promoting cervical cancer screening among Vietnamese American women. *American Journal of Public Health, 97*(9), 1693–1700.

National Association of County Health Officers (NACCHO). 2014. *Public health experience with health disparities: Community health worker program, Erie County Health Department, Ohio.* Washington, DC.

Navarro, A.M., R. Raman, L.J. McNicholas, and O. Loza. 2007. Diffusion of cancer education information through a Latino community health advisor program. *Preventative Medicine, 45*(2–3), 135–138.

Nelson, K.A., G. Highstein, J. Garbutt, K. Trinkaus, E.B. Fisher, S.R. Smith, and R. Strunk. 2011. A randomized controlled trial of parental asthma coaching to improve outcomes among urban minority children. *Archives of Pediatric and Adolescent Medicine, 165*(6), 520–526.

Nelson, K.A., G. Highstein, J. Garbutt, K. Trinkaus, S.R. Smith, and R.C. Strunk. 2012. Factors associated with attaining coaching goals during an intervention to improve child asthma care. *Contemporary Clinical Trials, 33*(5), 912–919.

Olson, E.C., G. Van Wye, B. Kerker, L. Thorpe, and T.R. Frieden. 2006. *Take Care Inwood and Washington Heights. NYC Community health profiles, Second Edition. 19*(42), 1–16. New York City Department of Health and Mental HygieneNew York City, NY.

Nguyen, T-U., J. Tran, M. Kagawa-Singer, and M.A. Foo. 2011. A qualitative assessment of community-based breast health navigation services for Southeast Asian women in southern California: Recommendations for developing a navigator training program. *American Journal of Public Health, 101*, 87–93.

Nuno, T., M.E. Martinez, R. Harris, and F. Garcia. 2011. A promotora-administered group education intervention to promote breast and cervical cancer screening in a rural community along the US-Mexico border: A randomized controlled trial. *Cancer Causes and Control, 22*, 367–374.

O'Brien, M.J., A.P. Squires, R.A. Bixby, and S.C. Larson. 2009. Role development of community health workers: An examination of selection and training processes in the intervention literature. *American Journal of Preventive Medicine, 37*(6, Supplement 1), S262–S269.

O'Neill, K., K.J. Williams, and V. Reznik. 2008. Engaging Latino residents to build a healthier community in mid-city San Diego. *American Journal of of Preventive Medicine, 34*(3S), S36–S46.

Ockene, I.S., T.L. Tellez, M.C. Rosal, G.W. Reed, J. Mordes, P.A. Merriam, . . . Y. Ma. 2012. Outcomes of a Latino community-based intervention for the prevention of diabetes: The Lawrence Latino Diabetes Prevention Project. *American Journal of Public Health, 102*(2), 336–342.

Olds, D.L., J. Robinson, R. O'Brien, D.W. Luckey, L.M. Pettitt, C.R. Henderson, Jr., . . . A. Talmi. 2002. Home visiting by paraprofessionals and by nurses: A randomized, controlled trial. *Pediatrics, 110*(3), 486–496.

Olds, D.L., J. Robinson, L. Pettitt, D.W. Luckey, J. Holmberg, R.K. Ng, . . . C.R. Henderson, Jr. 2004. Effects of home visits by paraprofessionals and by nurses: Age 4 follow-up results of a randomized trial. *Pediatrics, 114*(6), 1560–1568.

Ornelas, I., E. Eng, and K. Perreira. 2011. Perceived barriers to opportunity and their relation to substance use among Latino immigrant men. *Journal of Behavioral Medicine, 34*(3), 182–191.

Ortman, J.M., and C. Guarneri. 2010. *United States population projections*. US Bureau of the Census, Department of Commerce, Suitland, MD: US Government Printing Office.

Otero-Sabogal, R., D. Arretz, S. Siebold, E. Hallen, R. Lee, A. Ketchel, . . . J. Newman. 2010. Physician-community health worker partnering to support diabetes self-management in primary care. *Quality in Primary Care, 18*(4), 363–372.

Palmas, W., J.A. Teresi, S. Findley, M. Mejia, M. Batista, J. Kong, . . . O. Carrasquillo. 2012. Protocol for the Northern Manhattan Diabetes Community Outreach Project. A randomised trial of a community health worker intervention to improve diabetes care in Hispanic adults. *BMJ Open, 2*(2), e001051.

Panchanadeswaran, S., and B.A. Dawson. 2011. How discrimination and stress affects self-esteem among Dominican immigrant women: An exploratory study. *Social Work in Public Health, 26*(1), 60–77.

Passel, J.S., and D.V. Cohn. 2009. *A portrait of unauthorized immigrants in the United States*. Washington, DC: Pew Research Center.

Pati, S., and S. Danagoulian. 2008. Immigrant children's reliance on public health insurance in the wake of immigration reform. *American Journal of Public Health, 98*(11), 2004–2010.

Peers for Progress. 2014. Sustainable financing for peer support within reach: Funding models for community health workers. In *Peer support around the world* (pp. 1–3). Washington, DC: American Academy of Family Practice Physicians Foundation.

Percac-Lima, S., J. Ashburner, B. Bond, S. Oo, and S. Atlas. 2013. Decreasing disparities in breast cancer screening in refugee women using culturally tailored patient navigation. *Journal of General Internal Medicine, 28*(11), 1463–1468.

Peretz, P., L. Matiz, S. Findley, M. Lizardo, D. Evans, and M. McCord. 2012. Community health workers as drivers of a successful community-based disease management initiative. *American Journal of of Public Health, 102*(8), 1443–1446.

Perez, L.M., and J. Martinez. 2008. Community health workers: Social justice and policy advocates for community health and well-being. *American Journal of Public Health, 98*(1), 11–14.

Perez-Escamilla, R. 2011. Acculturation, nutrition, and health disparities in Latinos. *American Journal of Clinical Nutrition, 93*(5), 1163S–1167S.

Perry, H.B., R. Zulliger, and M.M. Rogers. 2014. Community health workers in low-, middle-, and high-income countries: An overview of their history, recent evolution, and current effectiveness. *Annual Review of Public Health, 35*, 399–421.

Perumalswami, P.V., S.H. Factor, L. Kapelusznik, S.L. Friedman, C.Q. Pan, C. Chang, . . . D.T. Dieterich. 2013. Hepatitis Outreach Network: A practical strategy for hepatitis screening with linkage to care in foreign-born communities. *Journal of Hepatology, 58*(5), 890–897.

Philis-Tsimikas, A., A. Fortmann, L. Lleva-Ocana, C. Walker, and L.C. Gallo. 2011. Peer-led diabetes education programs in high-risk MexicanAmericans improve glycemic control compared with standard approaches: A Project Dulce Promotora randomized trial. *Diabetes Care, 34*, 1926–1931.

Philis-Tsimikas, A., C. Walker, and L. Rivard. 2004. Improvement in diabetes care of underinsured patients enrolled in project dulce: A community-based, culturally appropriate, nurse case management and peer education diabetes care model. *Diabetes Care, 27*(1), 110–115.

Postma, J., C. Karr, and G. Kieckhefer. 2009. Community health workers and environmental interventions for children with asthma: A systematic review. *Journal of Asthma, 46*(6), 564–576.

Prezio, E.A., D. Cheng, B.A. Balasubramanian, K. Shuval, D.E. Kendzor, and D. Culica. 2013. Community Diabetes Education (CoDE) for uninsured Mexican Americans: A randomized controlled trial of a culturally tailored diabetes education and management program led by a community health worker. *Diabetes Research and Clinical Practice, 100*(1), 19–28.

Price, M., and L. Benton-Short. 2008. *Migrants to the metropolis: The rise of immigrant gateway cities*. Syracuse, NY: Syracuse University Press

Raich, P.C., E.M. Whitley, W. Thorland, P. Valverde, and D. Fairclough. 2012. Patient navigation improves cancer diagnostic resolution: An individually randomized clinical trial in an underserved population. *Cancer Epidemiology Biomarkers and Prevention, 21*(10), 1629–1638.

Ramirez, A., E. Perez-Stable, F. Penedo, G. Talavera, J.E. Carrillo, M. Fernández, . . . K. Gallion. 2014. Reducing time-to-treatment in underserved Latinas with breast cancer: The Six Cities Study. *Cancer, 120*(5), 752–760.

Ramos, R.L., J.B. Ferreira-Pinto, M.L. Rusch, and M.E. Ramos. 2010. Pasa la Voz (Spread the Word): Using women's social networks for HIV education and testing. *Public Health Reports, 125*, 528–533.

Renzaho, A.M., C. Gibbons, B. Swinburn, D. Jolley, and C. Burns. 2006. Obesity and undernutrition in sub-Saharan African immigrant and refugee children in Victoria, Australia. *Asia Pacific Journal of Clinical Nutrition, 15*(4), 482–490.

Romero, A.J., D. Martinez, and S.C. Carvajal. 2007. Bicultural stress and adolescent risk behaviors in a community sample of Latinos and non-Latino European Americans. *Ethnicity and Health, 12*(5), 443–463.

Rosenthal, E.J., N. Wiggins, J.N. Brownstein, S. Johnson, I.A. Borbon, and J.G. De Zapien. 1998. *Weaving the future: The Final report of the National Community Health Advisor Study*. Tucson: University of Arizona.

Rosenthal, E., J. Brownstein, C. Rush, G. Hirsch, A. Willaert, J. Scott, . . . D. Fox. 2010. Community health workers: Part of the solution. *Health Affairs, 29*(7), 1338–1342.

Rosenthal, M.P., F.D. Butterfoss, L.J. Doctor, L.A. Gilmore, J.W. Krieger, J.R. Meurer, and I. Vega. 2006. The coalition process at work: Building care coordination models to control chronic disease. *Health Promotion Practice, 7*(2 Supplement), 117S–126S.

Rostila, M. 2010. Birds of a feather flock together—and fall ill? Migrant homophily and health in Sweden. *Sociology of Health and Illness*, *32*(3), 382–399.

Rothschild, S.K., M.A. Martin, S.M. Swider, C. Tumialan Lynas, I. Janssen, E. Avery, and L.H. Powell. 2013. Mexican American Trial of Community Health Workers: A randomized controlled trial of a community health worker intervention for Mexican Americans with type 2 diabetes mellitus. *American Journal of Public Health*, *104*(8), 1540–1548.

Ruggiero, L., S. Oros, and Y. Choi. 2011. Community-based translation of the Diabetes Prevention Program's lifestyle intervention in an underserved Latino population. *Diabetes Educator*, *37*(4), 564–572.

Ruiz, Y., S. Matos, S. Kapadia, N. Islam, A. Cusack, S. Kwong, and C. Trinh-Shevrin. 2012. Lessons learned from a community–academic initiative: The development of a core competency–based training for community–academic initiative community health workers. *American Journal of Public Health*, *102*(12), 2372–2379.

Saad-Harfouche, F.G., L. Jandorf, E. Gage, L.D. Thelemaque, J. Colon, A.G. Castillo, M. Trevino, and D.O. Erwin. 2011. Esperanza y Vida: Training lay health advisors and cancer survivors to promote breast and cervical cancer screening in Latinas. *Journal of Community Health*, *36*(3), 219–277.

Sable, M.R., J.D. Campbell, L.R. Schwarz, J. Brandt, and A. Dannerbeck. 2006. Male Hispanic immigrants talk about family planning. *Journal of Health Care for the Poor and Underserved*, *17*(2), 386–399.

Sale-Shaw, J. 2013. Community asthma control in NYC: Methods, outcomes and lessons learned. Presentation for *Asthma in New York City, New York City Asthma Partnership*. May, 2013. New York City: NYC DOHMH.

Salinero-Fort, M.Á., L. del Otero-Sanz, C. Martín-Madrazo, C. de Burgos-Lunar, R.M. Chico-Moraleja, B. Rodés-Soldevila, . . . P. Gómez-Campelo. 2011. The relationship between social support and selfreported health status in immigrants: An adjusted analysis in the Madrid Cross Sectional Study. *BMC Family Practice*, *12*(1), 46–54.

Sanchez, J., G. Silva-Suarez, C.A. Serna, and M. De La Rosa. 2012. The Latino Migrant Worker HIV Prevention Program: Building a community partnership through a community health worker training program. *Family and Community Health*, *35*(2), 139–146.

Shah, M., E. Kaselitz, and M. Heisler. 2013. The role of community health workers in diabetes: Update on current literature. *Current Diabetes Reports*, *13*(2), 163–171.

Siahpush, M., G. Heller, and G. Singh. 2005. Lower levels of occupation, income and education are strongly associated with a longer smoking duration: Multivariate results from the 2001 Australian National Drug Strategy Survey. *Public Health*, *119*(12), 1105–1110.

Siahpush, M., T.T. Huang, A. Sikora, M. Tibbits, R.A. Shaikh, and G.K. Singh. 2014. Prolonged financial stress predicts subsequent obesity: Results from a prospective study of an Australian national sample. *Obesity*, *22*(2), 616–621.

Siatkowski, A.A. 2007. Hispanic acculturation: A concept analysis. *Journal of Transcultural Nursing, 18*(4), 316–323.

Singh, G., M.D. Kogan, and S.M. Yu. 2009. Disparities in obesity and overweight prevalence among US immigrant chidlren and adolescents by generational status. *Journal of Community Health, 34,* 271–281.

Singh, G.K., and R.A. Hiatt. 2006. Trends and disparitites in socioeconomic and behavioural characteristics, life expectancy, and cause-specific mortality of native-born and foreign-born populations in the United States, 1979–2003. *International Journal of Epidemiology, 35,* 903–919.

Singh, G.K., and M. Siahpush. 2002. Ethnic-immigrant differentials in health behaviors, morbidity, and cause-specific mortality in the United States: An analysis of two national data bases. *Human Biology, 74*(1), 83–109.

Singh, G.K., S.M. Yu, M. Siahpush, and M.D. Kogan. 2008. High levels of physical inactivity and sedentary behaviors among US immigrant children and adolescents. *Archives of Pediatric and Adolescent Medicine, 162*(8), 756–763.

Singh, P., and CHW Technical Task Force. 2011. One million community health workers: Technical Task Force Report. The Earth Institute. New York, NY: Columbia University.

Spencer, M., J. Hawkins, N. Espitia, B. Sinco, T. Jennings, C. Lewis, . . . E. Kieffer. 2013. Influence of a community health worker intervention on mental health outcomes among low-income Latino and African American adults with type 2 diabetes. *Race and Social Problems, 5*(2), 137–146.

Spencer, M.S., A-M. Rosland, E.C. Kieffer, B.R. Sinco, M. Valerio, G. Palmisano, . . . M. Heisler. 2011. Effectiveness of a community health worker intervention among African American and Latino adults with type 2 diabetes: A randomized controlled trial. *American Journal of of Public Health, 101*(12), 2253–2260.

Stewart, M.J., A. Neufeld, M.J. Harrison, D. Spitzer, K. Hughes, and E. Makwarimba. 2006. Immigrant women family caregivers in Canada: Implications for policies and programmes in health and social sectors. *Health and Social Care in the Community, 14*(4), 329–340.

Stoddard, P. 2009. Risk of smoking initiation among Mexican immigrants before and after immigration to the United States. *Social Science and Medicine, 69*(1), 94–100.

Suter, E., J. Arndt, N. Arthur, J. Parboosingh, E. Taylor, and S. Deutschlander. 2009. Role understanding and effective communication as core competencies for collaborative practice. *Journal of Interprofessional Care, 23*(1), 41–51.

Tang, T.S., M. Funnell, B. Sinco, G. Piatt, G. Palmisano, M.S. Spencer, . . . M. Heisler. 2014. Comparative effectiveness of peer leaders and community health workers in diabetes self-management support: Results of a randomized controlled trial. *Diabetes Care, 37*(6), 1525–1534.

Taylor, V.M., T.G. Hislop, S.P. Tu, C. Teh, E. Acorda, M.P. Yip, . . . Y. Yasui. 2009. Evaluation of a hepatitis B lay health worker intervention for Chinese Americans and Canadians. *Journal Community Health, 34*(3), 165–172.

Thimot, J., A. Martinez, and S. Matos. 2004. No soft money!—A model sustainable health outreach program. Presented at the American Public Health Association Annual Meeting, *November 2004*.

Thompson, J.R., C. Horton, and C. Flores. 2007. Advancing diabetes self-management in the Mexican American population: A community health worker model in a primary care setting. *Diabetes Educator, 33*(Supplement 6), 159S–165S.

Thyne, S.M., and S.A. Fisher-Owens. 2011. The complexities of home visitation for children with asthma in underserved communities. *Journal of Asthma, 48*(2), 210.

Thyne, S.M., J.P. Rising, V. Legion, and M.B. Love. 2006. The Yes We Can Urban Asthma Partnership: A medical/social model for childhood asthma management. *Journal of Asthma, 43*(9), 667–673.

Torres, L., S.D. Yznaga, and K.M. Moore. 2011. Discrimination and Latino psychological distress: The moderating role of ethnic identity exploration and commitment. *American Journal of Orthopsychiatry, 81*(4), 526–534.

Tran, N., A. Portela, L. de Bernis, and K. Beek. 2014. Developing capacities of community health workers in sexual and reproductive, maternal, newborn, child, and adolescent health: A mapping and review of training resources. *PLoS One, 9*(4), e94948.

Uiters, E., W. Deville, M. Foets, P. Spreeuwenberg, and P.P. Groenewegen. 2009. Differences between immigrant and non-immigrant groups in the use of primary medical care; a systematic review. *BMC Health Services Research, 9*, 76.

United Nations Department of Economic and Social Affairs. 2011. *International migration report 2009: A global assessment*. New York, NY: United Nations.

United Nations Department of Economic and Social Affairs. 2013. *International migration policies: Government views and priorities*. New York, NY: United Nations.

US Department of Health and Human Services. 2007. *Community Health Worker National Workforce Study*. Bureau of Health Professions, Health Resources and Services AdministrationWashington, DC: US Dept. of Health and Human Services.

US Department of Homeland Security. 2013. *Yearbook of immigration statistics 2012*. Washington, DC: Author.

US Department of Labor. 2009. *Department of Labor 2010 Standard Occupation Classification. Federal Register, 74*(12), 3923.

US Department of Labor. 2014. Occupational employment and wages, May 2013:Community health workers. In *Occupational Employment Statistics*, No. 21 p. 1094. Washington, DC.

Venditti, E.M., and M.K. Kramer. 2013. Diabetes prevention program community outreach: Perspectives on lifestyle training and translation. *American Journal of Preventive Medicine, 44*(4, Supplement 4), S339–S345.

Vimo, J., and B. Weiner. 2013. *Maximizing health care reform for New York's immigrants*. New York Immigration Coalition. New York, NY: New York State Health Foundation,

Viruell-Fuentes, E.A. 2007. Beyond acculturation: Immigration, discrimination, and health research among Mexicans in the United States. *Social Science and Medicine*, 65(7), 1524–1535.

Viruell-Fuentes, E.A., P.Y. Miranda, and S. Abdulrahim. 2012. More than culture: Structural racism, intersectionality theory, and immigrant health. *Social Science and Medicine*, 75(12), 2099–2106.

Viswanathan, M., J. Kraschnewski, B. Nishikawa, L.C. Morgan, P. Thieda, A. Honeycutt, ... D. Jonas. 2009. Outcomes of community health worker interventions. *Evidence Report/Technology Assessment (Full Report)*, 181, 1–144, A141–142, B141–114, passim.

Vojta, D., T.B. Koehler, M. Longjohn, J.A. Lever, and N.F. Caputo. 2013. A coordinated national model for diabetes prevention: Linking health systems to an evidence-based community program. *American Journal of Preventive Medicine*, 44(4, Supplement 4), S301–S306.

Volkmann, K., and T. Castanares. 2011. Clinical community health workers: Linchpin of the medical home. *Journal of Ambulatory Care and Management*, 34(3), 221–233.

Walton, J.W., C. Snead, A. Collinsworth, and K. Schmidt. 2012. Reducing diabetes disparities through the implementation of a community health worker-led diabetes self-management education program. *Family and Community Health*, 35(2), 161–171.

Wells, K., M. Rivera, S. Proctor, G. Arroyo, S.A. Bynum, G.P. Quinn, ... C.D. Meade. 2012. Creating a patient navigation model to address cervical cancer disparities in a rural hispanic farmworker community. *Journal of Health Care for the Poor and Underserved*, 23(4), 1712–1718.

Wennerstrom, A. 2011. Community-based participatory development of a community health worker mental health outreach role to extend collaborative care in post-Katrina New Orleans. *Ethnicity and Disease*, 21(3 Supplement 1), 45–51.

Werner, D., and B. Bower. 2012. *Helping health workers learn*. San Francisco, CA: Hesperian Foundation.

Wiggins, N., D. Johnson, M. Avila, S.A. Farquhar, Y.L. Michael, T. Rios, and A. Lopez. 2009. Using popular education for community empowerment: Perspectives of community health workers in the Poder es Salud/Power for Health program. *Critical Public Health*, 19(1), 11–22.

Wingate, M.S., and G.R. Alexander. 2006. The healthy migrant theory: Variations in pregnancy outcomes among US-born migrants. *Social Science and Medicine*, 62(2), 491–498.

Wingood, G.M., R.J. DiClemente, K. Villamizar, D.L. Er, M. DaVarona, J. Taveras, ... R. Jean. 2011. Efficacy of a health educator-delivered HIV prevention intervention for Latina women: A randomized controlled trial. *American Journal of Public Health*, 101, 2245–2252.

Wolin, K., L. Colangelo, B. Chiu, and S. Gapstur. 2009. Obesity and immigration among Latina women. *Journal of Immigrant and Minority Health*, *11*(5), 428–431.

World Health Organization (WHO). 2011. *Health of migrants*. Paper presented at the 9th Coordination Meeting on International Migration. Geneva, Switzerland: WHO.

WHO. 2013. World Health Statistics 2013. Geneva, Switzerland.

Zsembik, B.A., and D. Fennell. 2005. Ethnic variation in health and the determinants of health among Latinos. *Social Science and Medicine*, *61*(1), 53–63.

Index

Page numbers in *italics* indicate figures and tables.